Parents and Their Deaf Children

Parents and Their Deaf Children

The Early Years

Kathryn P. Meadow-Orlans
Donna M. Mertens
Marilyn A. Sass-Lehrer

With contributions from
Kimberley Scott-Olson

Gallaudet University Press
Washington, D.C.

Gallaudet University Press

Washington, DC 20002

http://gupress.gallaudet.edu

Library of Congress Cataloging in Publication Data

Meadows-Orlans, Kathryn P.
   Parents and their deaf children: the early years / Kathryn P. Meadow-
Orlans, Donna M. Mertens, and Marilyn A. Sass-Lehrer; with contributions
from Kimberley Scott-Olson.
        p. cm.
   Presents research findings from surveys and interviews of parents conducted
by the National Parent Project (1996–2002).
   Includes bibliographical references and index.
   ISBN 1-56368-137-4
      1. Parents of deaf children—United States—Attitudes. 2. Deaf children
—Services for—United States—Evaluation. 3. Hearing impaired children
—Services for—United States—Evaluation. 4. Deaf children—Education—
United States—Evaluation. 5. Hearing impaired children—Education—
United States—Evaluation. 6. Deaf children—United States—Family rela-
tionships. 7. Hearing impaired children—United States—Family relation-
ships. 8. National Parent Project. I. Sass-Lehrer, Marilyn, 1948– II.
Mertens, Donna M. III. Title.

HV2551 .M43 2003
362.4'2'0830973—dc21
                                                        2002192763

♾ The paper used in this publication meets the minimum requirements of
   American National Standard for Information Sciences—Permanence of
   Paper for Printed Library Materials, ANSI Z39.48–1984.

Contents

Preface

Any research-based book has a large cast of characters to whom the authors are indebted, and this book is no exception. Our first debt of gratitude is to the parents who contributed their experiences with intervention services during their children's early years. More than 400 parents completed a questionnaire, and more than 80 were interviewed. Their enthusiastic participation was a motivating force. We salute their dedication to their children and thank them for their time and thoughtful contributions.

The Gallaudet Research Institute provided welcome financial support, and we appreciate the encouragement of Thomas Allen and Michael Karchmer. We are grateful for the contributions of four Gallaudet graduate students: Kimberley Scott-Olson (1996–1998; 2001), Selena Steinmetz (1997–1999), Jennifer Pittaway (1999–2001), and Susan Medina (2000–2001). The school personnel who organized focus groups must remain anonymous to protect the identity of the sites and participants, but they have our gratitude.

Members of Gallaudet's Center for Assessment and Demographic Studies were helpful in the survey phase: Thomas Allen, Brenda Rawlings, and Arthur Schildroth helped to design the questionnaire; Sue Hotto and Arthur Schildroth supplied information for program sampling.

We thank the following for their contributions to the survey instrument: Carl Dunst for permission to incorporate items from the Family Support Scale; Project Dakota for the use of items from a service-satisfaction scale; the Utah SKI★HI program for items from the Language Development Scale; Rita LaPorta and Karen Saulnier for assistance in development of the communication items; Barbara Raimondo and Leslie Proctor for providing parents' perspectives.

Kathryn Ritter-Brinton provided helpful comments on the book proposal. Rosaline Crawford, Arlene Stredler-Brown, and Ivey Pittle Wallace

(Gallaudet University Press) gave welcome suggestions on an earlier draft of the manuscript.

Several chapters incorporate interview material that appeared in a chapter by Mertens, Sass-Lehrer, and Scott-Olson, "Sensitivity in the Family-Professional Relationship: Parental Experiences in Families with Young Deaf and Hard of Hearing Children" (P. E. Spencer, C. J. Erting, & M. Marschark [Eds.], *The Deaf Child in the Family and at School: Essays in Honor of Kathryn P. Meadow-Orlans,* Mahwah, NJ: Erlbaum, 2000.) We have also included comments from attendees at national conferences where data from the project were presented.

The book is very much a team effort, with the three senior authors participating in planning and carrying out each phase of a complex effort. Meadow-Orlans coordinated the survey and took the lead for chapters 1, 3, 5, and 6. Mertens and Sass-Lehrer supervised the interviews and focus groups. Mertens took the lead in chapters 4, 7, and 8, and Sass-Lehrer, in chapters 2 and 9. Kimberley Scott-Olson contributed to many aspects of the data collection and coding and collaborated on chapter 7. Jennifer Pittaway helped to prepare the resources appendix.

Thanks to the chairs of two Gallaudet University departments for support during the years of our involvement in the National Parent Project: Barbara Bodner-Johnson (1996–1998) and Richard Lytle (1998–2002), Department of Education, and Thomas Kluwin, Department of Educational Foundations and Research.

We echo the thought of one parent participant: "I hope that it helps somebody else. I really hope it helps some other parent some day—that would make me feel really good."

Kathryn P. Meadow-Orlans
Donna M. Mertens
Marilyn A. Sass-Lehrer

Chapter 1
Introduction to the National Parent Project and Survey Results

This book details the experiences of a representative group of American parents and their deaf or hard of hearing children from identification of hearing loss to the early elementary grades during the last decade of the twentieth century. The parents report their goals and expectations, the children's achievements and troubles, their family's satisfactions and disappointments with health and educational systems. When the children were born, in 1989 and 1990, these systems were in the throes of dramatic shifts in provisions for infants and toddlers with disabilities. Technological advances led to the expanded use of cochlear implants and earlier identification of hearing loss. The Individuals with Disabilities Education Act (IDEA), passed in 1986 and reauthorized in 1997, required that parents be included in planning educational programs for their children with disabilities and that programs be designed to meet the needs of these children and their families (Craig, 1992; Moores, 2001; Sass-Lehrer & Bodner-Johnson, 1989).

However, if professionals are to provide individualized support services, they must first identify salient characteristics of families and children so the services will fit unique circumstances. This seems a straightforward statement, but it masks a complex imperative. Deaf and hard of hearing children comprise a heterogeneous population: They come from every region and state; from farms, inner cities, and suburbs; and from every racial, ethnic, and socioeconomic group. They may be adopted or fostered, have many siblings or none, and live in large or small extended families where parents speak English or one of many other languages. Those parents may be hearing, deaf, or hard of hearing; married or single, living with a partner, divorced, or separated. The children themselves may be deaf or hard of hearing, may or may not have additional conditions, and may or may not be developing at age level. All of these characteristics (and others as well) have an impact on the kinds of services that are most

1

appropriate, on parents' evaluations of services, and on parents' responses to a child's hearing loss.

To date, few efforts have been made on a national level to explore the relationship of child and parent characteristics to early intervention services. This gap was one reason for the National Parent Project (NPP), which is reported in this book. A nationwide survey was conducted that was designed to reach parents of 6- and 7-year-old deaf and hard of hearing children and to gather information about their early experiences with the professionals who provided identification and intervention services.[1] To gain an in-depth understanding of those experiences, the survey was followed by interviews with 80 of the parents.

A growing body of research documents the positive effects of early comprehensive intervention for the social and cognitive development of children born at risk for developmental delay (Greenberg & Crnic, 1988; Hauser-Cram, Warfield, Shonkoff, & Krauss, 2001; Shonkoff, Hauser-Cram, Krauss, & Upshur, 1992). For children who are deaf or hard of hearing, positive results of early intervention are shown for social and communicative competence, and support networks relate to positive mother-child interaction and better language development (Calderon & Greenberg, 1997; Meadow-Orlans & Steinberg, 1993; Yoshinaga-Itano, 2000). Children in responsive and supportive families demonstrate better socioemotional, communicative, and cognitive development compared to others (Meadow-Orlans, in press). A lingering question for practitioners is how best to connect with families to provide information, support, and resources to enhance parents' and caregivers' abilities to promote children's development. Professionals also face the challenge of changing demographics of children in special education programs (Holden-Pitt & Diaz, 1998; Schein, 1996). As immigration has increased the proportion of foreign-born children in public schools, nonnative children in deafness-specific programs have increased even more rapidly (Schildroth & Hotto, 1993), perhaps because economic disadvantage places them at greater risk

---

1. See Appendix A for a detailed description of the survey methodology. Appendix B includes the survey and interview instruments.

for repeated middle-ear infections and poor medical care (Cohen, Fischgrund, & Redding, 1990).

These demographic changes, added to legislative and technological shifts, mean that both early intervention programs and the children and families they serve are quite different from those of earlier years. Information about the composition of the population and about parents' views of their early experiences should benefit professionals and future consumers alike.

Design of the Project

The NPP was conducted in three stages: (1) a national survey of parents whose 6- and 7-year-old children were enrolled in educational programs for pupils who were deaf or hard of hearing (404 respondents); (2) telephone or TTY interviews with parents randomly selected from survey respondents who agreed to provide additional information (62 interviews); and (3) face-to-face interviews (one with an individual mother, one with a mother-father pair, and three in focus groups with a total of 17 mothers). Readers will find detailed descriptions of the research methodology in Appendix A and copies of the survey questionnaire and interview guides in Appendix B.

Parents of 6- and 7-year-old children were targeted for the following reasons: (1) All children with even a mild congenital hearing loss will probably be identified by age 6; (2) all of the children and parents would have had an opportunity to participate in (or would have failed to receive) intervention services; (3) a fairly narrow age span would increase the homogeneity of parental expectations for developmental progress; and (4) parents would be close enough in time to the infant and preschool years to provide accurate retrospective reports and also sufficiently removed to gain some perspective on those experiences.

Plan of the Book

The following pages of this introduction present the survey results, providing a broad snapshot of the characteristics of 6- and 7-year-old deaf and hard of hearing children and their parents, drawn from across the United

States. In addition, we have summarized the parents' assessments of early intervention services, their responses to their child's hearing loss, and their child's behavioral status and linguistic progress. The following chapter draws from comments from all of the parents, discussing their communication choices for their deaf and hard of hearing children. The next five chapters provide perspectives of parents from important subgroups: (1) children who are hard of hearing, (2) children with additional conditions, (3) children who have deaf parents, (4) children with cochlear implants, and (5) children from minority families. The final section includes two chapters with a general focus, again drawing on the advice from all of the parents (1) to other parents of deaf and hard of hearing children and (2) to the professionals who serve those children and their families.

Survey Results
Characteristics of the Children

Meadow-Orlans and Sass-Lehrer (1995) proposed that the following child and parent characteristics are especially relevant to the success of early intervention: a child's hearing level; age at identification; the presence or absence of additional conditions; and the parents' hearing status, racial/ethnic group membership, and educational level. Data from the NPP survey suggest that these characteristics are indeed related to parents' evaluations of services, the support they receive, their assessment of the impact of deafness on the family, and assessments of children's social behaviors and language progress.

Hearing Level

Forty-six percent of the children the NPP survey describes were identified as deaf: "can't understand speech, even with a hearing aid"; the remainder were identified as hard of hearing: "can understand speech when in a quiet room, with a hearing aid." Lengthy discussions led to the decision to use this functional definition rather than asking parents to report decibel levels or audiological categories (e.g., "mild" to "profound") because responses might be more reliable if categories were couched in everyday language. Also, the survey was designed to capture parents' perceptions of their children's auditory functioning.

Age at Identification and Intervention

The child's average age when parents suspected a hearing loss was 17 months. On average, hearing loss was confirmed at age 22 months (an elapsed time of 5 months between initial suspicion and confirmation). However, 31% of parents reported confirmation less than 1 month after the initial suspicion, and 4% waited 2 years or more. Degree of hearing loss greatly influenced the confirmation age: Children who are deaf had a confirmed identification on average at age 14.5 months; those described as hard of hearing had a confirmed identification at 28.6 months. Thus, children who are deaf received confirmation of hearing loss earlier than those born even a decade earlier. Time between parental suspicion and confirmation of hearing loss is within the expected range, confirming the guarded optimism that Harrison and Roush (1996) express—that age of identification is slowly decreasing. Also heartening are reports that implementation of newborn hearing screening in Colorado "has increased dramatically" the number of children identified before the age of 6 months (Yoshinaga-Itano, Sedey, Coulter, & Mehl, 1998).

Like age at identification, age at intervention varied greatly. Children who are hard of hearing began speech training 8 months after their hearing loss was identified; those who are deaf began training 11 months after identification.[2] Although the average time required for a child to receive a hearing aid was almost 8 months after identification, 20% of the children received a hearing aid within 1 month. One source of this variation is the children with deaf parents, who tend to delay procuring amplification. Children with deaf mothers got hearing aids at an average age of almost 19 months. Children with hearing mothers were exposed to sign language at differing ages, depending on the racial or ethnic background of their parents: White children at 9 months, Hispanic children at 15 months, and African American children at 19 months.[3]

---

2. Ages are rounded to the nearest month. Unless otherwise noted, reported group differences are statistically significant. Appendix C includes supplementary tables showing additional data. For ages at which deaf and hard of hearing children received hearing aids, speech and auditory training, sign language, and cued speech, see Appendix C, Table 1.

3. For the survey, parents checked their race or ethnicity as White, Hispanic, Black/African American, Asian Pacific, Native American, or Other.

Additional Conditions

Almost by definition, the needs of a child with a hearing loss are compounded by cognitive or physical disabilities (Meadow-Orlans, Smith-Gray, & Dyssegaard, 1995). Traditionally, approximately one third of school-age children who are deaf or hard of hearing are reported to have additional conditions (visual, cognitive, motor, or learning disabilities; health or behavioral problems) that may interfere with educational achievement (Schein, 1996). Parents participating in the NPP survey identified 32% of their children with some additional condition, although data from the annual survey of 6- and 7-year-olds conducted by the Center for Assessment and Demographic Studies (CADS) show that only 24% have additional conditions. However, CADS data (collected from program personnel rather than from parents) for children of all ages show that about one third have additional conditions (Wolff & Harkins, 1986; Schildroth & Hotto, 1993). It is possible that program personnel are reluctant to label children as young as 6 years, especially for conditions such as learning or developmental disabilities and emotional or behavioral problems. These data suggest that parents may be more likely than teachers to identify these conditions when their children are young.

Characteristics of Families

Hearing Status of Parents and Siblings

Among responding parents, 10% of mothers and 11% of fathers are deaf or hard of hearing. Ten hearing mothers are married to deaf (DF) or hard of hearing (HH) husbands; nine hearing fathers are married to DF or HH wives; 7.5% of the children have two DF or HH parents; 5.5% have one DF or HH parent. Eighteen percent of the children have no siblings; 3% have one deaf sibling only; and 79% have one or more hearing siblings.

Educational and Occupational Status

Parents' educational levels are moderately high: Some training beyond high school was reported by 39% of mothers and 31% of fathers; 27% of mothers and 33% of fathers have 4 years of college or more. More than half of the mothers (58%) work outside the home: 55% in professional or managerial positions, 32% in clerical or sales work, and 14% in blue-collar jobs. Fathers' occupations are described as professional or managerial (40%), clerical or sales (20%), or blue collar (40%).

Racial/Ethnic Background

The proportion of Whites in the survey data (67%) is somewhat higher than that reported for this age group (58%) in the CADS annual survey for 1996–1997 (Holden-Pitt & Diaz, 1998). However, the NPP distribution of Hispanic and African American respondents is somewhat different from that for the CADS annual survey. This might be partially attributed to schools' differing classifications of children from mixed-race families. CADS and NPP survey distributions are as follows: Hispanic (17% and 11%, respectively); African American (17% and 9%); Native American (1% and 1%); Asian/Pacific (3% and 3%); and mixed or other (2% and 9%). Mixed-race families were most likely to be African American-plus-White or Hispanic-plus-White.

Services Received

Special Services for Children

Parents identified, described, and evaluated the early intervention program that their child attended the "longest." Children who are deaf entered that program on average at age 29.5 months; those who are hard of hearing entered the program on average at age 34.5 months. Elapsed time after identification was 16 months for the deaf group and 11 months for the hard of hearing group.

About 60% of parents reported that they had more than one program to choose from. (Note that fully 40% of parents reported that they did *not* have a choice of programs for their child.) Of those who had a choice, 29% selected a program because sign language was offered as a communication approach; 12% chose the program because an oral approach was available. A few mentioned location, individual attention, availability of special services, and opportunity to be with other deaf children or to be included in programs with hearing children as decisive attributes. Of those who reported that they had no program choices, 80% either said that they preferred the program or gave no response to the question about preference. Four percent would have preferred a signing program; another 4%

would have preferred an oral program. Almost half (48%) reported that program staff included one or more deaf adults.[4]

In about one quarter of the programs, speech alone was the communication approach used; sign language plus speech was used in two thirds; sign language alone in 5%; cued speech in 3%; and sign language plus cues in 3%.

Services for Parents

Apparently, programs are doing a good job of providing relevant information to parents. Three quarters received information about deafness; 68% had information on legal rights for their children; 64% had information on child behavior and/or development; and 59% had information on choices for future school placement. Sign language instruction was available to 71% (and to 89% of parents whose children were enrolled in programs that used signs). About half of the fathers and three fourths of the mothers attended classes. Parent group meetings were available to 69% of the parents. Of those, 44% of fathers and 85% of mothers attended meetings. Individual counseling was available to 43% of families; 25% of fathers and 70% of mothers made use of those services. Parents identified the single service that was most helpful to them. About one third of mothers selected information about deafness, legal rights of children, child behavior or development, or school placement. Another third selected sign language instruction. Other responses were divided among several different categories. For 27% of the fathers, information was the most helpful; sign language instruction was the most helpful for 41% of the fathers.

Parents' Evaluations of Early Services

Most parents had positive evaluations of their services.[5] When we assigned scores from 1 to 4 to responses and summed these scores, the average score was 14 of a possible 16 points. Hearing mothers evaluated services significantly more positively than did mothers who are deaf or hard of hearing,

---

4. See Table 2 in Appendix C for tabular data on communication approach used in "first" and "current" educational programs and "at home" for all of the children and by hearing status.

5. Appendix C, Table 3.

and White mothers were more positive about services than mothers from non-White or mixed-race families.[6]

Neither the mothers' education (no college versus some college) nor the child's hearing status nor the presence of an additional condition affected service evaluation scores. However, the child's age at the time of identification was a significant factor in the evaluation of services by parents of non-White and mixed-race children, and older ages were associated with less positive evaluations.

Sources of Help for Parents

Thirteen potential sources of help for parents were listed, and parents indicated the helpfulness of each source.[7] Teachers received the highest score of any support source. Two thirds of parents characterized their child's teacher(s) as "extremely helpful"; an additional one quarter characterized a teacher as "very helpful." This compares with 47% and 20% for spouses and only 19% and 20% for medical doctors. Parents of children with additional conditions reported *less* support than parents of children whose deafness was not complicated by some disability. Non-White respondents and those with no college training reported less support than did other groups.[8]

Children's Behaviors and Language Ratings

Children's Behaviors

We asked parents to characterize their child's behavior by reacting to 10 behavioral descriptions, for example, "My child forms warm, close attachments to or friendships with peers."[9] A behavior score summarizing these items shows that (1) for children with no additional conditions, those who are deaf have more positive behaviors than those who are hard of hearing and that those with early diagnoses have more positive behaviors than those with late diagnoses; however, (2) for children with one or more

---

6. Appendix C, Table 4.
7. Appendix C, Table 5.
8. Appendix C, Table 6.
9. Appendix C, Table 7.

additional conditions, those who are hard of hearing have more positive behaviors than those who are deaf, and those with late diagnoses have more positive behaviors than those with early diagnoses.[10] Perhaps for children with other conditions, those whose hearing losses were diagnosed late had services related to another condition that supported their behavioral development. It appears that hard of hearing children with late diagnoses and no additional conditions may need special help during the preschool years.

Children from non-White or mixed-race families whose mothers have no college training are also at additional risk for behavior problems. Their behavior scores are significantly below those of other children.[11] This suggests that additional counseling resources would benefit parents and children in programs with high concentrations of less-educated minority families.

Language Ratings

As expected, hard of hearing children received significantly higher language scores than children who are deaf.[12] Age at identification and additional conditions also influence language performance. Children with one or more cognitive or physical conditions have lower scores than their peers without disabilities. For hard of hearing children without additional conditions, early identification is associated with higher language scores. For children with additional conditions, those with later diagnoses have significantly higher language scores regardless of whether they are deaf or hard of hearing. This result, which is counterintuitive but similar to that for behavioral problems, is puzzling and warrants further investigation.[13] The mother's education and racial/ethnic group are also related to language scores: White and non-White children with more highly educated mothers score higher than same-race peers whose mothers have less education.[14] Within educational levels, White children have higher language scores than non-White and mixed-race peers.

---

10. Appendix C, Table 8.
11. Appendix C, Table 9.
12. Table 10 in Appendix C shows these items in abbreviated form together with the proportions of children with the highest ratings.
13. Appendix C, Table 11.
14. Appendix C, Table 12.

Parents' Feelings about Deafness

Parents responded to nine statements designed to measure the impact of deafness on them and/or their families and registered agreement or disagreement on a five-point scale.[15] Parents of children with conditions in addition to deafness reported a significantly more negative impact compared to parents of children without additional conditions. Mothers' hearing status had a lesser but still significant influence on impact scores. A child's deafness had a less significant impact on deaf mothers than on hearing mothers. Parents' racial/ethnic background also influenced the impact scores: Hispanic mothers reported a more negative impact than White mothers.

Conclusion

Early intervention specialists may want to give special attention both to late-diagnosed children who are hard of hearing and to minority-group parents with less education. A report of interviews with Hispanic parents includes provocative insights into their attitudes, perceptions, and beliefs about deafness and contains important information for educators. Religious and cultural values influence families, some of whom attribute deafness to divine will and experience the stigmatization of a deaf child by the extended family (Steinberg, Davila, Collazo, Loew, & Fischgrund, 1997). Demographers predict that the current population trend toward smaller proportions of non–Hispanic and larger proportions of Hispanics and African Americans in the U.S. population will continue at least until 2050 (Hernandez, 1997). This forecast adds urgency to the challenge of meeting the needs of children and families from minority backgrounds.

The interview data presented in the following chapters provide important views of parents and are intended to flesh out the less personal information available from a statistical analysis of data derived from a survey questionnaire.[16]

---

15. Table 13 in Appendix C lists these statements with the mean score for each item.

16. Many of the data reported in this chapter appeared previously in *American Annals of the Deaf* (1997, 142, 278–293).

Chapter 2
Communication Conundrum: Family Solutions

Within the first day after we found out, I knew I had to start signing with her because . . . nobody could tell me whether she'd ever be able to hear enough to learn how to talk, and I didn't want a frustrated child or—or me. So it was a real easy decision. I didn't even think twice about it. (Survey 293)

[He] was already learning speech . . . and [we wanted him to] keep going with it—being oral. He has some hearing; he has some residual hearing; he's already speaking. He wants to speak. "Do it!" It wasn't even a decision. It was made for me rather than me making one. I never even thought of sign language, to be honest with you. Unless he was going to go totally deaf and then, you know, obviously I was going to have to go sign language. (Survey 76)[1]

Communication is the central concern for families with children who are deaf and hard of hearing. Parents struggle to establish effective communication in their families and ensure that their children receive the necessary support from schools and professionals. Early language acquisition and child and family functioning, regardless of the mode of communication, are critical to the overall development of the child with a hearing loss. However, parents and professionals may lose sight of this as they grapple with a decision. Recognizing the vital importance of effective com-

---

1. Survey forms were numbered consecutively from 1 to 404 when they were received at Gallaudet. Numbers were also used to identify the interviewees. They are retained here merely to reflect the large number of different respondents included as sources. Excerpts from focus groups are also identified by a sequential numbering system.

munication between families and children, researchers have studied the relationship between various methods of communication, child language outcomes, academic achievement, and social development (Calderon & Greenberg, 1997; Carney & Moeller, 1998; Desselle, 1994; Geers & Moog, 1992; Greenberg, Calderon, & Kusché, 1984; Lynas, 1999; Meadow-Orlans, 1987; Vacarri & Marschark, 1997; Yoshinaga-Itano, 2000).[2] Communication mode and parent-child interactions have also been the subject of numerous investigations (Calderon & Greenberg, 1997), and research has more recently focused on the quality of communication and overall family functioning (Rosenbaum, 2000). Despite efforts to determine the best mode of communication for children with hearing loss, definitive answers remain elusive (Carney & Moeller, 1998).

Early attempts to determine the most appropriate communication approach were based on a system that weighted factors such as degree of hearing loss and presence of additional conditions (Downs, 1974; Geers & Moog, 1987). Stredler-Brown (1998) suggests that professionals can make recommendations based on a data-driven approach utilizing assessment protocols that focus on the child's development and parent-child interactions, along with consideration of parent preference. Attempts to reduce the decision to an objective, quantifiable measure that minimizes the importance of subjective variables that influence parental choices may have limited success. In a recent study of factors contributing to parents' selection of a communication mode, Eleweke and Rodda (2000) find that decisions are heavily influenced by the information parents receive, perceptions of the effectiveness of assistive technology, attitudes of service professionals, and the quality and availability of support services. Steinberg and Bain (2001) conclude from interviews with 30 families that communication decisions are based as

---

2. See the following websites and books for a description of the different modes of communication that people who are deaf or hard of hearing commonly use: http://www.beginningssvcs.com; http://clerccenter.gallaudet.edu/SupportServices/series/4010.html; *Choices in Deafness: A Parent's Guide to Communication Options* (2nd edition), Sue Schwartz (Ed.); *The Silent Garden: Raising Your Deaf Child* (2nd edition), by Paul W. Ogden.

much on child and parent characteristics as they are on the information and guidance that professionals provide and the availability and quality of services. Parental knowledge, experiences, and personalities influenced the communication decisions of one family who participated in Spencer's in-depth study (2000a). Kluwin and Gaustad (1991) suggest that attitudes about hearing loss, acceptance of a child with a disability, and parental expectations for the child's role in the family influence the family's communication decision. Decisions are often complicated by perceived time pressures, that is, the need to develop early language, the ability to understand complicated information, and the parents' emotional state (Steinberg & Bain, 2001). Steinberg and Bain interviewed families whose children's hearing losses were identified by 6 months of age. These families discussed the impact of accuracy, completeness, and timeliness of information, as well as support they received.

The National Parent Project (NPP) asked parents to describe the communication approaches they used with their children at home and in school and their involvement in the communication choices they made. Parents shared their perspectives on how communication decisions were managed in the early years and their satisfaction with the process. Parents identified the method of communication used at home, in an early intervention program before age 5 years, and in their child's current program (Table 2 in Appendix C).

The parents' hearing status greatly influences their choice of methodology. Parents who are deaf are more likely to sign at home with their children than hearing parents regardless of whether their children are deaf or hard of hearing. However, differences are also based on the extent of the child's hearing loss. For example, 57% of hearing parents and 40% of nonhearing parents with hard of hearing children use speech only at home with their child. On the other hand, only 9% of hearing parents and no parents who are deaf or hard of hearing use speech only if their child is deaf. In early intervention programs, speech plus sign language was the approach used most frequently with all of the children. As children moved from early intervention to elementary school, some parents reported that their children's method of communication changed from sign language plus speech to either sign language without speech, speech without signs, or Cued Speech. Overall, very few children in this study used Cued Speech or an auditory verbal approach.[3]

One mother described the change of communication mode over time with her hard of hearing daughter:

They suggested having her learn some basic signing skills when she was a baby because we didn't know exactly how she would develop behaviorally with a hearing loss. We did start that, and we talked about other means of communication like Cued Speech. We kind of went through all of that and then it became apparent that she was developing orally. We subsequently stopped doing any kind of signing with Helen whatsoever because she . . . is doing well verbally. She's on target at the average 2½ years old for speech. (Survey 297)

Another parent had this to say about a child's early communication needs:

The child needs to be in a signing environment, especially at a young age. That is their communication, that is their vocabulary . . . that is the foundation. . . . How they're gonna learn when they get older? . . . [You] can make the choices as to how that child's progressing. . . . You can make your choices later on, but . . . when they're young they need to be in a signing environment, and I suggest a deaf school. (Survey 288)

---

3. The auditory verbal approach emphasizes the development of listening skills through one-on-one therapy that focuses attention on the use of the remaining hearing (with the aid of amplification). Because this method strives to make the most of a child's listening abilities, no manual communication is used and the child is discouraged from relying on visual cues, including speechreading. The main goal of this unisensory approach is to develop speech, primarily through the use of aided hearing alone, and the communication skills necessary for integration into the hearing community (http://www.beginningssvcs.com/communication_options/auditory_verbal.htm).

The Communication Decision

Parents utilize many different strategies to determine the communication method to use with their children. Some families have strong opinions and make decisions early with little or no input from professionals. Others struggle as they attempt to reconcile the information they receive from professionals that conflicts with their own beliefs or with the opinions of others. Many parents emphasize a desire for their children to be able to communicate with both hearing and nonhearing people. Still, some parents describe a sense of relief when they believe that their child's speech has improved to the point where they do not need sign language to communicate. Some families receive little information or support and are on their own in making a decision.

Parents consider communication options an important factor in the selection of an early intervention program. Parents who could choose an early intervention program reported that they chose a particular one mainly because of the communication approach it offered. Nearly half of the parents had no program choice, and some would have preferred another program because of the limited communication options available. Twenty-five percent reported that the early intervention program did not offer a choice in the communication approach it used.

For some parents, the communication decision is second nature. All of the deaf parents whom we interviewed used at least some sign language with their children and described their decisions as fairly straightforward. Many used American Sign Language (ASL), whereas others used a combination of speech and signs incorporating English word order or signs from English-based sign systems.[4] For example, one deaf mother with a deaf son explained why she chose to use sign language:

---

4. American Sign Language is a complete signed language with distinct grammatical rules, word order, and idioms. It is the primary language of many Deaf people in the United States. Signed English systems are manually coded systems that use signs from ASL and invented signs for spoken English words, prefixes, and endings. Signed English systems are not languages but are used to support spoken English. Examples of Signed English systems are Seeing Essential English (SEE I), Signing Exact English (SEE II), and Signed English.

Well, it [sign language] is just our natural language. Sometimes I use some English, I would say pidgin language. (Survey 316)

Some of the hearing parents we interviewed were also quite sure from the beginning about the communication mode they would use. A few parents had very strong feelings about their child's need to get along in the "hearing world." One parent said:

The majority of the world is a hearing world, a speech world, and . . . if she's signing to people . . . you know, most of them are not gonna under- stand what she's trying to say. . . . Once we realized she was gonna hear . . . you know, we were really pushing that, you know, that she'd be oral. I mean, had she not been as successful as she has been, you know, I guess we would've . . . you know, fallen back on the sign. (Survey 101)

One father who chose a combined approach (i.e., signing and speech) considered the need to get along in the hearing world but was also influ- enced by his experiences with Deaf adults in his church:

Well, I think at least for me it's a pretty simple decision. I feel that . . . I want her to learn to read lips, I want her to speak. . . . But I see how well adjusted these adults are that can read lips, that can sign, and that have some vocal ability. And in the hearing world in the job market, when you're an adult . . . as a parent, for Sabrina's future, I don't . . . see any other way other than Total Communication. . . . I don't believe in bury- ing her in the Deaf culture and not teaching her to get along in a hearing world and have her just be with deaf people and just her own kind. I don't think the world's like that. . . . We need to learn with our abilities or dis- abilities. . . . So that's my view on Total Communication. I'm pretty adamant on that and I don't feel there's any other, any other way. (Survey 310)

Fear of "losing your child to the Deaf culture" is another concern of some parents:

If you just stuck with sign, my thinking was, he's locked in this Deaf World . . . and I decided he would have to fit into both worlds. And I told him when he was real little, once he had a hearing aid on . . . and when he heard me when I would get real close and be talking to him I'd say "We're gonna cross over and you're gonna fit into our world because I'm not gonna let go. . . . God gave you to me. . . . I'm hanging on tight. You're stuck; you're not getting away." (Survey 16)

Some parents based their decisions on how much hearing their child had. An ear, nose, and throat specialist told one father that his daughter was able to hear at a normal conversational level, although background noise was a significant problem. Because she was "able to hear almost everything," these parents decided to use speech only (Survey 85). Another parent said:

He has no hearing at all. . . . I can't use just speech with him . . . because I have to communicate with him. . . . I have to communicate with my son. And my whole household, my husband, and my 3-year-old daughter . . . we all sign with him. But we also use voice, and he . . . tries to make sounds, but it doesn't sound like anything. (Survey 17)

Several parents indicated that they wanted to ensure that their children had every opportunity to use whatever mode of communication would work for them. Spencer (2000a) describes one family who explored all of the communication options for their daughter. By their daughter's first birthday they were using an English-based sign system and Cued Speech, each for half of the day, to promote bilingualism. At 2 years of age they agreed to drop Cued Speech and focus on signing. By the time their daughter was 3 years old, they had decided on a cochlear implant, resting their hopes on improved auditory and speech skills. They continued to use signs after the implant and were hopeful that these avenues would be sufficient for her to develop literacy (see chapter 6). Several parents in the NPP expressed a similar desire for their child to have everything. One Spanish-speaking mother with a deaf son shared these thoughts with a focus group:

What I was thinking is, there's lipreading, speechreading, and sign—the whole 9 yards. So they can have an option, you know, if they grow up and they said, "Oh, I don't want to sign," or "I just want to speak," that's their choice. But I want to give them some options; it's what you can do, you know. So they gave us some speech therapies at home, and they integrate much more speech in their classroom. And we got him [an] auditory FM system. (Focus Group 2)

Other mothers had similar responses:

Because we want him to have opportunity and every advantage . . . so [you] know, we don't care; we just want him to learn. We want him to be able to talk; we want him to be able to communicate; and we want to be able to communicate with him. And if that means signing, that's what we're [going to] do. (Survey 334)

Well, I wanted Derick to learn. I wanted him to use all means of communication. Whatever it was to be able to communicate. So I couldn't make that choice—one over the other. It was, like, cues, voice, and oral, and visual. . . . Communication means so much to me. My background is social work, and that's what you say. People have to talk, you have to communicate—use any means necessary. (Focus Group 3)

Some families expressed anguish about their decisions and wondered whether they had made the right ones. A discussion from one of the focus groups illustrates this struggle:

Parent 6: You know, it's really just trial by error. You happened to put him in a program that benefited him. You could have went and not benefited from being in an oral program. You might have had to make another decision down the line.

Parent 1: Right. [We] could have bottomed out. The thing is you don't know if your decision is right or wrong . . .

Parent 6: There's no right or wrong. There's no answer. It's a guessing game until you die. (Focus Group 3)

Advice from Professionals

Despite the literature that emphasizes the importance of presenting all of the communication options and collaborative decision making (Moeller & Condon, 1994; Stredler-Brown, 1998), many families were told by professionals which approach would be best for their child. In some cases, these parents did not realize that choices existed. One mother described how Total Communication was selected for her son:

When we went to [school] they kind of stressed that. They kind of stressed the fact that he needs all, every, all the communication. You know he don't need to learn just one thing. He needs to learn everything that he can. Don't limit him—that's basically what they said. . . . I'm open to anything that's gonna help him be better . . . and get along better. Of course there's nothing else offered, but, you know, whatever the school says . . . would make it easier for him, I'm willing to do. (Survey 202)

Complicating the decision for many families are the strong, sometimes biased, opinions among professionals about what is "right" for the child who is deaf. Regardless of whether one is advocating sign language or oralism, ardent views on communication methodology can put parents on the horns of a dilemma and be counterproductive to the decision-making process. In an influential paper on the failure of the education of deaf children, Johnson, Liddell, and Erting (1989) proposed that American Sign Language be the language of instruction for all deaf children. Low achievement levels, according to these authors, are the result of the lack of access to ASL and low expectations by professionals. Lane, Hoffmeister, and Bahan (1996) suggest that hearing parents who communicate with their child only through spoken English may be limiting the child's ability to acquire language, stunting cognitive development, damaging the parent-child relationship, creating tension among family members and frustration for the deaf child, or hindering social and emotional development.

A parent of twin boys described this conflict:

> As I'm sure you're aware . . . each agency thinks that their methodology is the best. And that they try to shove that down your throat. . . . Our thought as hearing parents was, "Oh, let's give 'em Total Communication; this will work really well." . . . It was appealing from a hearing standpoint, but when you started paying attention to what the Deaf community had to say about it and children who are being raised by Deaf parents, it's different, and ASL is a much more natural means of communication, and that's ultimately what we've chosen. And now we're starting to break off into some SEE [Signing Exact English] just for the benefits of, you know, reading and writing . . . and you wouldn't believe the flack we've caught from that. (Survey 348)

Equally one sided are the opinions of proponents of an oral approach who suggest that most children with hearing losses have sufficient residual hearing, with appropriate amplification to acquire language through listening (Ling, 1989; Lynas, 1999). They may tell parents that reliance on sign language will inhibit a child's motivation to learn to speak and interfere with the child's ability to attend to the "weaker" auditory signal. One parent encountered a speech therapist with very strong opinions about the use of sign language:

I had one speech therapist who basically accused me, told me, I was doing a total disservice by even, like, exposing Diana to sign language because she had so much hearing and her speech was so good. You know, that she shouldn't even be exposed to sign and I was saying, but yeah, she has all of this hearing now, but what if she doesn't have any in 5 years? Then what is she supposed to do? (Survey 75)

Parents are sometimes told that sign language is easier for deaf children and therefore their children may not accept the more difficult challenge of learning to speechread and talk. One mother said that professionals told her that if her daughter signed she would never talk and sign language would be her only mode of communication. This family ultimately found an oral program that accepted profoundly deaf children because, in her words, "the lady that told us [about the sign language program] saying that she'll never speak scared me to death" (Survey 226). Another mother said, "Well, we talked to some people who . . . advised us not to teach her sign language. And that if she did sign, she wouldn't speak" (Survey 30).

The following comment describes the bias of some professionals:

It just seems to me that there's so many people, you know, that have in their own mind what is the right way to educate or the right method of communication and that's part of what they're trying to pass on to parents . . . instead of making something available and saying, "OK, these are the things that are available, these are the things that are used, and this is where you can find out about them." . . . I mean, I wouldn't have known, like, Cued Speech. I wouldn't have known it had existed if I hadn't read about it first. (Survey 75)

Although many parents complained of professionals who presented conflicting information or had personal biases, others found that they were on their own to investigate the available options. Wolfe (2001) interviewed

25 families from rural areas of Georgia, Kentucky, Louisiana, North Carolina, and Tennessee about educational decisions for children who were deaf or hard of hearing. She found that many families had limited information or choices and often had to depend upon themselves to gather information. One NPP parent was not aware that there were choices available until she met another parent with a child who was deaf:

> I didn't know my options or anything so I got him into sign language with a deaf teacher who was oral because she was postlingually deaf when she was 11 . . . and she started teaching him a little sign language. . . . In the meantime I met a woman . . . and her son was oral and he had a severe-to-profound loss. . . . She showed me films of . . . the baby sitting around, and this child could speak really, really well. And . . . I showed her my son's audiogram, and she said your son should do better since he has more hearing than my son. So we got into the auditory verbal program . . . and the biggest help was [name of professional] . . . because she kinda explained that a child is like a computer and you have to program it. Keep on talking and keep on encouraging the child to listen and hear, and it will pay off, and it took 7 or 8 years, but it has. (Survey 286)

Comparisons between children, especially by extent of hearing loss, are a common but ineffective way to determine which communication approach to use. Many factors affect a child's ability to use residual hearing to acquire language and develop clear speech (Yoshinaga-Itano & Sedey, 2000).

Choosing Sign Language

We asked parents who chose to sign with their children why they had chosen this approach. Some parents commented on the importance of an early language foundation:

> I don't think it's fair for a kid who can't hear to use oral only. . . . I don't think you can start out that way. I think you have to start out with the

language base, the sign language, and then as the kid develops these audi-
tory skills and all that, you can kinda see how they're doing and maybe at
times go in and out, depending on what the situation is. (Survey 293)

Another commented that she did not want to wait for her child to
develop language:

Everybody except for [the person who worked with the strict oral pro-
gram] suggested that sign language was appropriate and acceptable. It
was out in the world, too—sign language was more accepted. . . . We
wanted something that had a 100% guarantee method of success, and
sign language was the only guaranteed method. We wanted immediate
success. . . . And what I kept hearing was that pursuing the oral method
without any reliance on signs was so time intensive it might take months
and months before your child uttered a sound. My child was only 3
months old and her loss was so profound. . . . Sign was my success route.
It was never to the exclusion of giving her every opportunity to develop
speech. (Focus Group 1)

Another mother who was convinced that sign language was right for
her son explained it this way:

We never gave it a second thought. I had read the book Choices
[Schwartz, 1996], but I always felt signing was the way though I didn't
know the difference between Signed English and ASL. It's up to him. If he
wants to stop signing when he grows up, that's OK. (Focus Group 1)

Some parents do not understand that American Sign Language is a
complete language, equivalent in form and function to English. Other parents are confused about the differences between ASL and signed English
systems. One mother who researched the options said the following:

*We were conflicted with Signed English. Parents need to be better edu-
cated, and teachers need to be better able to explain the two. I simply
learned about both, but I did start with Signed English because English is
my native language, but I never could get the hang of all those prefixes
and suffixes, and my articles were thrown out the window immediately,
so it really turned into a pidgin sign, and soon after I stopped the initial-
izing as well. It's still very pidgin, but it's more toward ASL. It will be a
lifetime of learning. I will try to keep ahead of her.* (Focus Group 1)

Choosing Not to Sign

Several parents said that their children did not need sign language. Some
started out with signs but then stopped when their children began to
speak. One mother described using some Cued Speech to help her
daughter distinguish sounds such as "tah" and "dah." However, after
cochlear implant surgery she no longer needed cues.[5] This mother had
considered using sign language before the surgery but had decided
against it:

*The [cochlear implant] people we worked with . . . told us that it's bet-
ter not to use sign language if she's going to rely on the cochlear implant.
So at some point we may do that. At some point we may certainly let her
exercise the choice to learn sign language. But right now that would not
be compatible with her cochlear implant as we understand it, and she
communicates very well. The speech therapist is ready to let her out of
speech therapy.* (Survey 224)

Parents whose children were not profoundly deaf were often advised to
try speech first:

---

5. Professionals and parents disagree about the efficacy of the use of sign language prior
to and/or following cochlear implant surgery.

*[The day after the hearing loss was identified, when he was almost 3]
they got him into the early intervention program. They thought because
he has a hearing loss somewhere around 60 dB that he could go into the
auditory program. . . . [Interviewer: Did you ever consider using either
Cued Speech or signs?] No-o-o. We thought we'd try the auditory method
and see if it would work. And if it didn't work, then we'd go and try something else.* (Interview 1)

Another issue for parents is the perceived difficulty of learning to sign
(Luterman, 1999; Lynas, 1999). When asked why she and her husband had
chosen an oral approach with their daughter, one mother responded:

*To tell you the truth . . . we were so scared. . . . We didn't know sign,
either. And it would be like trying to teach somebody French when you don't
know French yourself. You know? And we just thought, well, this is what we
have to do. That is what, you know, we have to start learning it, we have
to start teaching it to her, but that is when I thought only, only if you had
some hearing could you go into a speaking program. . . . I mean it made me
much more relaxed to say OK, I already know how to talk. I can do this. . . .
So that's why . . . we really never did [sign].* (Survey 226)

Communication in the Family

The effectiveness of communication between parent and child appears to
have a more significant impact on a child's overall development than does
the particular form or method of communication they use. Effective parent-child communication is positively linked to language development,
academic achievement, early reading, social adjustment, and family functioning (Calderon, 2000; Desselle, 1994; Paul & Quigley, 1990; Marschark,
1997; Ritter-Brinton & Stewart, 1992; Rosenbaum, 2000). For the survey,
parents described communication used at home, satisfaction with their
child's language progress, and their child's language skills. We found no significant correlations between home communication and the child's language skills or parent satisfaction when the child's hearing level was con-

trolled. Mothers with more education reported better language for their children than mothers with less education.

Families generally used the same communication method at home as their children used at school. However, more families used speech alone at home (33% at home compared with 27% at school). Three of four of the parents surveyed reported that they used at least some sign language at home with their children. Even parents whose children were primarily oral and who encouraged their children to use speech at home used sign language as a way to clarify communication that was unclear. Families with children with cochlear implants used a range of communication strategies, including signs, to reinforce their children's listening and speaking skills. The communication in these homes varied depending upon the benefit the child received from the implant and the specific situation or visual or listening environment. The extensive use of signs with young children is in marked contrast to the situation 30 years ago when more than 90% of hearing parents used speech alone to communicate with their children (Marschark, 1997).

Speech-Only Homes

One third of all of the parents we surveyed said speech alone was the communication method they used the most with their child at home (56% with hard of hearing children but only 9% with deaf children). However, parents were not averse to the use of signs from time to time if they believed it was necessary:

> *We do not sign at home. Although my younger kids do know some of it. We just don't. She does so well with hearing aids and the lipreading and with her own speech that we just don't use it. You know, I said if she had to use it, it'd be different, but I know that she can use her voice. Well, I prefer her to use her voice. I would go with sign. . . . Even people that don't know she's got a hearing loss, they can understand what she's saying. . . . So I don't rely on it as a first, as the first way of communication. I rely on it here in the home as a backup if there's an area where Kathy . . . doesn't exactly catch what you are saying to her or what's being asked of her.* (Survey 211)

Another parent explained how the family uses signs:

It's pretty much speech now. . . . I mean . . . she understands, and to us, she hears pretty good, so I mean . . . she may ask us, "What, what?" every once in awhile, and if I don't feel like she understands, then I do sign with her, but basically we just use speech with her. (Survey 66)

Signing Homes

Only 10% of the parents said they use signs alone at home most of the time to communicate with their child. Although several families expressed a desire to provide a fully signing home environment, they often found that it was impractical to sign all of the time. One hearing parent who characterized the family as excellent signers described the challenges:

As best we can . . . we sign all of the time. And we do our best to make it an ASL sign. But because we have hearing children and hearing friends in and out a lot of times, it's more of a pidgin English—trying to match our spoken word to explain to our hearing nonsigning friends what we're signing to our son. . . . When our deaf friends come over then all of us just shut up our voices, and it becomes an ASL household.[6] (Survey 218)

This same family described how they ensure that signing is used at home:

We do have a rule. Anytime you're in the kitchen you must be signing. Anytime we're in there, it is absolute; we do our best in the other areas of the house to be signing, but 100% of the time you're in the kitchen, you must be signing. (Survey 218)

---

6. Pidgin Sign English, sometimes called pidgin English or contact signing, is a form of signed communication that follows the rules and patterns of the user's first language (e.g., English for hearing parents). Signs generally follow English word order, but signers also incorporate ASL idioms and facial expressions.

Another parent whose child attended a bilingual program that emphasized ASL as the primary mode of communication talked about the discrepancy between home and school communication:

We use ASL, and I talk when I sign, but they [the school] don't like it when I talk and sign. If I go down there, they would prefer that I close my mouth. But I do like to use my mouth when he's at home. That helps for him to understand and . . . formulate mouth movements—kind of . . . lipread a little bit. We write and we have closed-caption TV, so he's learning to read and everything where he can start to read and communicate with me, but basically we sign. (Survey 53)

The deaf parents we interviewed generally use ASL as the primary language in the home. However, several parents reported codeswitching from ASL to contact sign.

Signing and Speaking Homes

The parents we interviewed who use both speech and signs at home cited the importance of access to communication for everyone in the home as their primary rationale for using the "Total Communication" approach. Others believe that by using speech they will increase their child's exposure to English and speechreading. Young (1997) interviewed 12 parents/caregivers of deaf children who were enrolled in a bilingual early intervention program and discovered that these families mix spoken English and sign language for the same reasons. Parents in the NPP described how they actually implement the Total Communication approach at home:[7]

---

7. The bilingual intervention program provided regular weekly visits with the family and made available hearing teachers who focused on communication strategies, implications of deafness, counseling, and collaboration with audiological, educational, and social services. In addition, weekly visits from Deaf adults focused on visual communication strategies, sign language instruction, and the abilities and achievements of Deaf adults. Both Deaf and hearing professionals provided weekly preschool classes for children and information sessions for families.

I sign and speak and sometimes just sign. It depends on the situation, and mostly at home we use pidgin. You know, when we're reading a story, if she's reading it for school, we'll do English; if they're trying to teach her the words, if she's getting graded on that book or something. But if I'm telling her a story or reading her a story, I try to use as much expression; I try to use more towards ASL [as much as] possible. (Survey 317)

Hearing siblings who have limited signing skills or who do not like to sign cause parents to modify the approaches they use at home. One parent said:

My oldest son hates to use it [sign language] for some reason. I don't know why he doesn't like to use it, but . . . [we] know he understands it, he just doesn't like to use it. I guess [be]cause it takes him so long to get things out. He sounds like a robot [chuckles]. By that time, Nathan is just going, "Would you hurry up, please?" (Survey 334)

Parent Communication Skills

We asked the parents who use sign language with their children to evaluate their own skills and those of others who have a significant role in their child's life. Only one third reported that both mother and father have either good or excellent signing skills. An additional one third reported that at least one parent has good or excellent signing skills. Although mothers and fathers rated their skill levels as the same in two out of three situations, the mothers' skills were the same as or better than the fathers' skills 95% of the time. This finding is consistent with those of other studies (Calderon and Low, 1998; Gregory, 1995; Kluwin & Gaustad, 1991; Meadow-Orlans, 1990) that indicate that mothers typically have better communication skills than fathers and often are disproportionately responsible for ensuring clear communication within the family.

Many parents talked about the difficulty of learning to sign. Courses and instructors were not always available or convenient. Many parents relied upon tapes, books, and even their children to teach them to sign:

We speak and sign at the same time. I obviously was not fluent in sign at the beginning, and I'm kind of learning . . . through classes, through books, through videotapes . . . the last couple of years. . . . My sign has grown with Sandra; we've learned together. I'd ask her a sign, she'll tell me the sign, we'll kind of learn it together, and I'm growing at the pace that she's growing. And our family is growing at that pace. We . . . always sign to her. I can't say the house is a 100%-sign house, where we always sign to each other whether she's around or not—because we don't, we speak. (Survey 310)

Another parent said:

We were still floundering; no [sign language] classes were offered, and we were also torn between Signed English and ASL. We didn't know—I was at a loss. You just can't learn on your own. You can't ask a child that age, "What's the sign for that?" (Focus Group 1)

Learning to sign was not easy for many families we interviewed. One family struggled initially with ASL, but by the time their son was 7 years old the whole family was signing:

The ASL was very hard for us. . . . Some of us couldn't grasp it right away. . . . [Now] the whole family is a fluent signer. We'll find that when it's something that we have to explain like really in detail and get into it, we turn off our voices and we sign only; but . . . we also speak to him, too, trying not to sign so that he can [get] a variety of different ways. But if we really have to get to the nitty-gritty with communicating with him, it would be ASL. (Survey 37)

Some parents who were successful in learning to sign attribute their skills to Deaf adults, some of whom are parents that they met through an early intervention program. Deaf adults serve as language and role models

in some early education programs, enhancing the communication skills of
hearing parents (Mohay, 2000; Watkins, Pittman, & Walden, 1998):

> *Interviewer: Who or what was the most helpful to you while you were
> there [name of early intervention program]?*

> *Parent: To me, I think the other parents. . . . They were very supportive.
> A lot of them were Deaf parents. I learned to sign from most of those
> parents. . . . I've never taken a course, or I had started one . . . in
> [name of state] and didn't finish it because we moved, but, you know,
> just the support system was wonderful.* (Survey 288)

Families with young children are less concerned about strict adherence
to a particular communication approach than they are about the practical
and functional aspects of communication in a family that has both deaf
and hearing members. Families frequently codeswitch from ASL to
English-based sign systems to speech. The home communication environment is flexible, marked by changes over time as children develop and
families acquire new information and develop new skills and as the practical need for different strategies in different situations arises.

Communication at School

Parents in the NPP enrolled their children in a wide variety of programs
including special preschool programs for children with developmental disabilities, programs affiliated with a school for deaf children, and local public schools. Within these settings, children were either in classrooms with
deaf and hard of hearing children only or in classrooms with hearing children. A few of the children had interpreters in their first-grade classes.
Most, however, were in programs with teachers or classroom aides who
were able to communicate directly with them. Several parents indicated
that they selected the program because of the communication approach
that it used. Finding an appropriate program that would meet their child's
needs was not always easy:

We did finally get in contact with the right people, and they had . . . serv-
ices provided for him in the local area school. But you know . . . the more
we found out, they just weren't providing [the] sign language [he need-
ed]. So we . . . finally made the decision to send him to the [state school
for deaf children] for the more appropriate services he needed. . . . I real-
ly don't think that they were . . . you know, equipped with the right peo-
ple to do this . . . [at the local area school]. . . . They weren't familiar
with the deaf. And . . . we had our go-rounds with 'em and it . . . was
just locking horns too much . . . and when we took a tour of the [state]
deaf school and became familiar with everybody and was told the servic-
es he'd be receiving . . . we knew that was the place for him. (Survey 231)

In general, parents were satisfied with the services they received from
their child's program. One parent thought that because of the school, her
son was ready to "face the world" and felt good about himself. Others
commented that because of the school program their children were able
to communicate, and they themselves were able to communicate with
their children. When the interviewer asked one mother what it was that
she liked so much about her daughter's program, she replied:

Well, you know, they were very helpful; they . . . helped us to learn to
communicate with Kyra, and they're just very [personable]. . . . They
just worked hard with us . . . and Kyra, she was signing. . . . Gosh, she
was signing her first words very quickly. (Survey 57)

In some instances the school placed more emphasis on speech than the
parents did at home, and the parents liked that. One parent described the
school for deaf children that her son was attending as "excellent": "They
worked with him. . . . They did things to increase his speech, they gave us
stuff to do at home" (Survey 185).

Another parent said:

It [speech] was working well with him . . . in the classroom and, you
know, his teacher, we communicate quite often with her. . . . She would

tell us some of the things—the words that he was having some problems with, mixing up his f's and s's and that kind of thing and so we just kind of . . . made sure to work with him a little on that . . . and even just in our daily language we try to use those specific words more often or to be sure and tell him . . . it's not . . . this, it's that. . . . I mean instantly, it was amazing how quickly . . . how well he did. (Survey 21)

The parents appreciated programs that were flexible in their communication approach and provided options:

That was the unique part about the [name of the program]. They had oral, they had TC. And if you were not making [it], [if] you felt you weren't making the right choice, you didn't have to disrupt everything to have him switch from one to the other. (Focus Group 3)

Communication Concerns

How am I going to communicate with my child? How will my child communicate with others? Will my child talk? These were the concerns of most of the interviewed parents:

I think the biggest [concern] was whether she'd learn to talk or not. And that was probably . . . underlying most of it for me. I'm sure my husband had some different ones. Of course, I was concerned about how to communicate. I bet that was, that was probably my biggest concern, was how do I communicate with my child. 'Cuz I can't imagine not being able to, you know. (Survey 317)

Two mothers shared these worries:

Could anything be done at all? Would he ever speak at all? Would he have, you know, a chance to be like any other kid? . . . Is he gonna have a fair chance? . . . What can we do to help him? (Survey 372)

Worrying about if he was going to be able to talk; worrying about how he was going to be accepted by other people, just basically worried about him. How . . . he was gonna make out in the world—you know, that can be cruel at times, and . . . I guess . . . my main concern was how it was going to affect him. (Survey 185)

Another mother focused on the importance of good communication with her daughter—not on her hearing loss:

Main fear: not being able to communicate because I know that communication is essential to any relationship. NOT "She won't be able to hear music"—much more basic. (Focus Group 1)

Some expressed the fear that their child might not be able to communicate with others—even in emergency situations. Difficulty communicating with other family members was especially painful for some parents:

Yeah . . . it's when your kid can communicate better with people you don't know or . . . people outside of the family more than people inside the family . . . you begin to wonder . . . especially grandkids . . . I mean, it's your grandkid, you should be able to communicate with him and not stare at him like you don't know what they're saying. (Survey 251)

Learning sign language and being able to keep up with their child's communication development was a common concern. One father whose child was enrolled in a program at a school for deaf children said:

It's like a never-ending battle. I guess, the older they get, the more they learn, and if you don't keep up with them, you fall behind. If you fall behind, they're going to continue learning. They're here all day. They're here from 8:30 to 2:30. . . . They're going to be here learning, and as they get older they're going to learn more and more. And you have to learn with them. . . . That's what it comes out to. You have to keep up with them because the kids learn fast at that age. . . . They're young, we're older. They pick it up faster. (Interview)

Although many of the initial concerns about communication had been lightened by their children's and their own communication progress, some parents still wondered whether the communication approach they had chosen was the best for their child.

Conclusion

Families identify communication choice as one of the most stressful decisions they have to make. Lack of information and resources or biased, incomplete, and inaccurate information from professionals makes the decision even more difficult. Families who are satisfied with their choices report that they had a lot of information on which to base their decision as well as support from professionals. Families struggling to make appropriate decisions may find *My Time to Learn: A Communication Guide for Parents of Deaf or Hard of Hearing Children* helpful (Figure 2-1). The developers of this checklist suggest that parents monitor their child's communication progress by considering these questions every 3 to 8 months. Parents may also want to consult the resources that Appendix D lists.

Although a decision about the best mode of communication may take time, parent-child relationships and language acquisition cannot be sacrificed or put on hold. Effective communication—signed, spoken, cued, or a combination—is vital to the quality of family life and to the child's emotional adjustment, language development, and future academic achievement.

Families are more concerned about getting the message across than about communication philosophies (Christiansen & Leigh, 2002; Young, 1997). Practical situations—in the car, at the dinner table, in mixed hearing and deaf groups—influence communication practices regardless of the "official" choice. Professional controversies and pressure to select an approach before parents understand the differences among methodologies

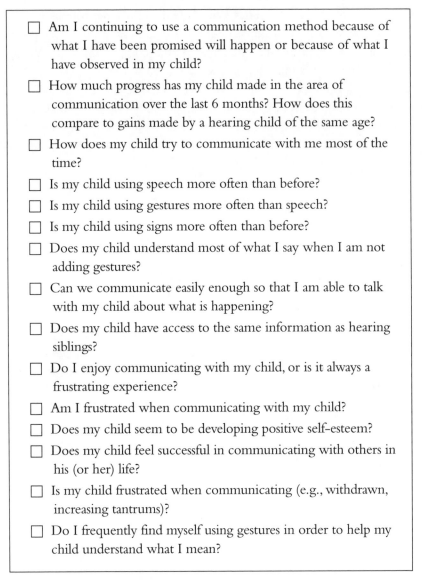

- [ ] Am I continuing to use a communication method because of what I have been promised will happen or because of what I have observed in my child?
- [ ] How much progress has my child made in the area of communication over the last 6 months? How does this compare to gains made by a hearing child of the same age?
- [ ] How does my child try to communicate with me most of the time?
- [ ] Is my child using speech more often than before?
- [ ] Is my child using gestures more often than speech?
- [ ] Is my child using signs more often than before?
- [ ] Does my child understand most of what I say when I am not adding gestures?
- [ ] Can we communicate easily enough so that I am able to talk with my child about what is happening?
- [ ] Does my child have access to the same information as hearing siblings?
- [ ] Do I enjoy communicating with my child, or is it always a frustrating experience?
- [ ] Am I frustrated when communicating with my child?
- [ ] Does my child seem to be developing positive self-esteem?
- [ ] Does my child feel successful in communicating with others in his (or her) life?
- [ ] Is my child frustrated when communicating (e.g., withdrawn, increasing tantrums)?
- [ ] Do I frequently find myself using gestures in order to help my child understand what I mean?

Figure 2-1. Family communication self-evaluation. From *My Turn to Learn: A Communication Guide for Parents of Deaf or Hard of Hearing Children* (S. Lane, L. Bell, & T. Parson-Tylka. Elks Family Hearing Resource Centre, Surrey, British Columbia, 1997).

or know their children's abilities exacerbate the difficulties parents experience with the decision-making process. Development of English language
skills or understandable speech influences the communication strategies
that most hearing families use. Many parents do not achieve the sign fluency they would like but use signs nevertheless to clarify messages and
reduce communication frustration. Because parents want their children to
have every opportunity, they do whatever they can to achieve this goal.

Chapter 3
Hard of Hearing Children: Forgotten and Overlooked

[Professionals] don't see a lot of kids with moderate losses. So Betsy was misdiagnosed really for years. Which has been very difficult for all of us.
(Survey 344)

Children with mild and moderate hearing losses were called "forgotten" almost a quarter of a century ago (Davis, 1977). In a revised edition of Davis's book, the editor notes that, in the years since the initial publication, "there has been a surge of both interest in and knowledge about children with mild to severe hearing losses," but despite dramatic improvements in identification, "the provision of appropriate educational and remedial services has not kept pace" (Davis, 1990, p. 1). One observer remarks that these children "are not so much 'forgotten' as they are overlooked" (Ross, 1990, p. 3). The disheartening experiences of many parents with hard of hearing children interviewed for the NPP suggest that many of their hearing losses were both overlooked and neglected.[1] In addition to describing the circumstances of the identification of their child's hearing loss and their reactions, the parents discussed their behavioral concerns, management of hearing aids, choice of communication mode, services they received, and their considerable coping skills.

---

1. Eighteen of the 40 parents randomly selected from the survey respondents who agreed to be interviewed had hard of hearing children. One mother was hard of hearing, and all of the fathers were hearing. In 13 families, both parents were White; in 2, both parents were African American. Three families included parents from two races. Eight of the children were boys; 10, girls. Four girls and two boys had conditions in addition to hearing loss.

Circumstances of Identification

The mother quoted at the beginning of this chapter believes that professionals see fewer children with mild or moderate losses, compared to the greater number of children with severe and profound losses, contributing to identification delays for such children. It is more likely that the symptoms of hard of hearing children are more difficult to assess because their apparent ability to hear varies in different environments and with different speakers. Prevalence figures show that mild or minimal hearing loss is more widespread than a more severe loss. Although profound deafness is estimated to occur in about 1 in 1,000 children (Schein, 1996), the prevalence of mild to moderate losses (26–70 dB) is estimated at 16 per 1,000, and some degree of reduced hearing in one or both ears is reported to be present in about 50 per 1,000 children (Bess, 1985). One group of researchers reports the prevalence of hearing loss among children ages 6 to 19 to be 7.1% (or 71 per 1,000). They include those with unilateral as well as bilateral losses and those with a 16-dB loss rather than the customary 26 dB, reasoning that children with these minimal losses also need special services (Niskar, Kieszak, Holmes, Esteban, Rubin, & Brody, 1998).

One family illustrates how children with a mild or moderate loss may escape identification for long periods, even when the family is observant and their medical care is excellent:

Yes, we knew something was wrong. But her hearing loss is moderate, and it's conductive, and she got to be very good at reading lips. So she would look like she's doing something else, and I'd say something to her, and she knew enough to look at me but then ask me again. Like say, "What?" But then by the time we finally got it diagnosed she had been through 13 other hearing tests. Some technicians thought she was, you know, within the normal range. And I think it's just difficult to test young children. . . . She got her hearing aids finally when she was 4. . . . We had her though in a special program offered by the school district where she had been tested. And you have to be two standard deviations below a mean on certain points before they'll let you into the special program, and she certainly was. Her tests were not geared for the hearing impaired, but it was clear she had difficulty with her speech, very clear. And so they allowed her into the program. So she . . . had already started speech therapy. But even when I told her speech therapist, . . . she said, "Really? She's hearing impaired?" . . . It's just an odd thing, I guess, with kids who are moderate. Sometimes it's even more difficult to tell what it is. (Survey 344)

This child illustrates a case of extreme identification delay. Her ability to speechread and to understand speech combined with her moderate hearing loss undoubtedly made identification more difficult. Nevertheless, a 2-year delay is both unusual and an understandable source of parental concern about professional services.

Another child's high-frequency hearing loss in both ears was not identified until he was 5 years old, even though his speech was delayed and his mother suspected the hearing loss when he was 3 years old. He, too, became proficient at speechreading, but his mother believes an additional factor was at work with him:

The preschool did have a hearing test, but because my son was so shy, they didn't push it. [They said,] "Oh well, he really doesn't want to do it, so it's OK." So they could have caught it there. And [the doctor] tested the hearing by just talking to him. (Survey 186)

Thus a delay in the identification of a hard of hearing child may be prolonged by personality traits associated with a reticence to being tested, by a teacher's reluctance or inability to overcome test resistance, or by inappropriate diagnostic methods.

Timely Identification with Little Parental Trauma

Although the survey data indicate that the experiences of these two families with late-identified hard of hearing children was the norm and not the exception, there was much variation in the diagnostic histories of children in this group. The age at identification ranged from 1 month to 72 months. The following example illustrates a case of early identification:

> *Alice was tested at birth because she weighed under 5 pounds. And [the hearing loss] was confirmed when she was 2 months old. . . . We took her to the hospital. The first time was in the hospital where I delivered her, and the second test was at Children's Hospital in [name of city].* (Survey 24)

In 1989, when this child was born, there was no automatic hearing screening. Some hospitals or pediatricians ordered screening for children with known risk factors: those with low birthweights (like Alice), those with family histories of hearing loss, or those with pre-, peri-, or postnatal trauma (Diefendorf, 1988).

An increasing number of states have enacted legislation providing universal newborn hearing screening (UNHS), and still others are screening on a voluntary basis. In May 2002, 65% of hospitals had instituted UNHS programs (National Center for Hearing Assessment and Management, 2002). It has been shown that universal screening leads to earlier identification and intervention, especially for children with moderate to profound losses, and that early intervention is associated with accelerated language development (Yoshinaga-Itano, Sedey, Coulter, & Mehl, 1998). The parent who related the following account experienced the difference that newborn screening can make. Her two daughters were both identified with a mild hearing loss:

> *My first daughter, Gail, is the oldest child. . . . She must have been about 3 years old when I noticed her starting to ask a lot to have things repeated. I was a little concerned, but I thought it was probably just a habit or a stage she was going through, always saying, "What? What?" . . . Then when she went to her 4-year-old well-child test, she failed her hearing screen a couple of times, and then subsequent testing [showed] she did have a mild-to-severe hearing loss in the right ear and a sloping moderate-to-severe loss in the left ear. . . . Helen is my third child. . . . She's*

about 2½ years old now. Because our hospital is working under a grant to test the efficacy of newborn hearing screening, she was screened at birth, at day two of her life. . . . They found [a hearing loss] right then, by one of those otoacoustic emissions tests, and they followed up [with an] ABR showing that she had a very similar loss to what Gail has. . . . She was fitted for hearing aids at about 5 months, and I think from the time she was 4 or 5 months we had a teacher of the hearing impaired come into our home once a week for an hour. . . . About 1½ years ago we started having speech therapists come into the home about once a month to work with her, [and now] those services have increased to once a week. (Survey 297)

The contrast in services provided to the two sisters is instructive, supporting the advantages of universal newborn hearing screening. However, it would be a mistake to believe the screening process will not miss any children or that these procedures protect children who lose their hearing after birth. Otitis media is one condition that continues to be a significant cause of hearing loss in children during the preschool years.

Hearing Loss After Birth: The Case of Otitis Media

Recurrent ear infections can cause either fluctuating or permanent conductive (usually less than profound) hearing loss (Roland, 1995). This condition, "otitis media with effusion," is sometimes referred to as "glue ear" (Wills, 1998). Children born with a cleft palate are more prone to repeated ear infections, as are members of some racial groups (Native Americans and Eskimos), those with frequent upper-respiratory infections, and those exposed to heavy tobacco smoke (Todd, 1986). The auditory effects of repeated infections are more likely to appear if the infections occur between the ages of 6 and 12 months, and episodes are likely to disappear or greatly decrease by 3 years of age. Some observers believe that the ill effects of conductive hearing loss will increase in the future because more young infants are being placed in day care centers, where infections are frequent (Downs, 1995).

Two parents described their child's recurrent ear infections. The first infection produced a mild high-frequency hearing loss, identified when the child was 4 years old:

> *He had a lot of ear infections as a baby, had his first set of tubes put in his ears when he was 9 months old. . . . The doctor asked us when we went in for his 6-month checkup if he did a lot of babbling, and we said, "Gee, you know, really, no, he doesn't." And so he checked that and found there was some fluid [in his ears]. Then they put the tubes in, and then he had a second set when he was 2 years old and another set right before he turned 4 and another set when he was [almost 6].* (Survey 21)

Another high-frequency hearing loss was identified when the child was 5 years old:

> *He had a lot of ear infections. Why did I first suspect his hearing loss? Because we knew he was developmentally slow in speaking. I remember asking the doctor if it could be related to his ear infections, and the doctor said, "No, he can hear." One of the main reasons we more aggressively pursued this was his babysitter could tell he was slow in speaking, and she started to push him more into talking. He would cry, he wouldn't want to go to her house.* (Survey 186)

Although the ear infections no longer recurred, the child continued to suffer from some of the social effects of these early experiences.

Response to Suspicion or Identification of Hearing Loss

Acceptance of Misdiagnosis

Two mothers illustrate how parents can be quick to accept a physician's false assurance of hearing acuity, even when their own observations suggest otherwise. The next mother believes that the misdiagnosis supported her hope that no hearing loss was present, attesting that parents are only too happy to accept good news:

> *The otolaryngologists in our area . . . looked me in the face and said, "It is not a hearing problem. I can look right at her and talk, ask a question, and it's obvious she can hear me." . . . Of course, I and my husband would much prefer if that weren't it. So it's easy to stay in denial if you don't have the support of a doctor. . . . Those blocks of 6 months really knocked a couple of years off [of her] ability to get a head start on her speech, and those early years are so critical. . . . I don't know what they [the doctors] were schooled in, but I still can't believe to this day that it took us 2 years, basically, from the time she was 2 until she was 4.*
> (Survey 344)

Another mother persisted in contacts with a pediatrician, even though her husband was happy to accept a misdiagnosis:

> *When he was 8 months old I took him to California to my best friend's house. . . . She said, "He's not responding." . . . She took a pan and a spoon and hit it behind his head, and he never flinched. . . . I took him right home, brought him over to the clinic where I worked and asked the pediatrician, who ran him through the auditory testing. He tested normal, quote unquote for an 8-month-old baby. . . . [Later on] he was making noises, humming tunes, but the words weren't coming out. It was "tookie" [instead of "cookie"]. He had his own language. By now he's 2½, almost 3. . . . I went to my pediatrician again, and I said, "Listen, he sounds like he's got marbles in his mouth." . . . It was hard to test him, but they did find a loss. But it took almost 2 years before I put my finger on it, saying "We gotta do something." But my husband was in denial: "There's nothing wrong with him, he's a normal kid, he'll grow out of it." That's what every parent in the world says, "He'll grow out of it."*
> (Survey 76)

Stress and Grief

Families understandably grieve at the news that a child has some condition with a far-reaching impact. Much has been written about the stress and chronic sorrow that parents of children with hearing loss express (Luterman, 1987; Koester & Meadow-Orlans, 1990; Meadow-Orlans, 1990; Moses, 1985). It is logical to imagine that parents with hard of hearing children might view that diagnosis as less serious than do parents whose children are deaf and that stress might therefore be less protracted. However, when survey responses are compared on the nine items that measure family stress related to hearing loss, parents with deaf children and those with hard of hearing children have scores that are no different except for the three items specific to communication. On these items, parents with HH children have more positive scores (e.g., "Much stress in my family is related to my child's hearing loss" versus "My child is regularly included in family conversations because we have an effective communication system"). The following excerpts from parent interviews provide further evidence that degree of loss does not lessen parental distress:

> [Initially] you're just overwhelmed, and you're kind of devastated, almost like you're in this despair and you don't have anybody to talk to or find out anything. So it makes it real tough. (Survey 66)

> We first found out that he was hard of hearing, 45% loss, in October, right before his third birthday. And I was devastated, absolutely devastated. And by Thanksgiving, he had all the [ear]molds made up for him, and by Christmas he was wearing hearing aids. He was then at 80% loss. So his was a progressive loss. Uhmm, I was like petrified. I'm going to end up with a deaf kid. I don't understand why. What's happening here? (Survey 76)

> I remember when we first found out—well, it's still difficult now. But I think at the time, one of the valuable things I did get from the materials I read . . . was that it is really like stages of grief. I do believe that and I personally found that [was true]. . . . Seek as much support as you can, learn as much as you can, and keep going. The child is still the same per-

son they were the day before you found out. And everything will fall into place. (Survey 344)

Acceptance: Focus on the Positive

Some parents cope with the stressful aspects of identification by focusing on the positive aspects of the situation, including the fact that the child has a mild or moderate rather than a profound loss or that no other physical or sensory conditions have been identified. However, this coping strategy can have a negative effect if parents use it to suppress the grief that is appropriate for the loss of the expected "perfect child." One clinician has observed that some families who use this strategy at the time of identification are less able to put grieving behind them and to use those energies for the concrete tasks of managing hearing loss (Harvey, 1989). At least for some parents, a focus on the positive has been helpful, as the following examples illustrate:

It helped me to focus on all that he had and not what he did not have, so I didn't fall apart. I knew that he could see, he could run, he could jump . . . and with hearing aids he could lead a normal life. So I guess when the shock comes that your child somehow doesn't have what the others have, I focused on what he does have . . . and it helped me put it in perspective. . . . Otherwise if all you dwell on is the disability, you can take it way out of proportion and think it's such a tragedy, or you don't get strong yourself or think some God-awful things are going to happen to this child and then we're not equipped to help him. (Survey 242)

Initially, [with my first child, Gail] not enough was done to explain it to me: why that was happening and if there are any other options. I just felt like they said, "OK, well, she's got this hearing loss, the only thing we can do is give her hearing aids." That was really hard for me to accept. And it was certainly easier with Helen because we knew so much more. But that was a very very difficult time for us, just emotionally when Gail's hearing loss was diagnosed . . . because it was so unexpected. (Survey 297)

Response to Identification of Hearing Loss: Guilt and Blame

"Almost all mothers of deaf children feel, at some level, that they are responsible for their child's deafness" (Luterman, 1987, p. 43). Luterman believes that parents who feel guilty are more likely to prolong the search for the cause of a hearing loss and to blame professionals for their inability to provide that information; instead, their energies could be put to better use in managing the hearing loss. The following interview examples show some of the directions that parents may take when they are beset by feelings of guilt and blame, which, in one case, is self-blame:

> I felt guilty because I had been, I guess, punishing her for not listening or not responding, but she really didn't hear me. (Survey 111)

> I guess my big thing was I blamed myself for not knowing until such a late age. . . . After I did all my crying and my blaming—wanting somebody else to blame—I sat down and thought, "This isn't good for Kathy to see me so upset about it. Because if she sees me upset and bothered by her hearing loss, it's going to bother her that she has a hearing loss." (Survey 211)

> I was a new mom. I didn't know. I should have really jumped on it earlier when he was 8 months old and listened more carefully. (Survey 76)

As the next example shows, delayed identification can also have unhappy and dramatic consequences for the child. This boy was described earlier as a child whose high-frequency hearing loss, suspected by parents when he was 3 years old, was not identified until he was 5½:

> The damage [done by delayed identification] was to his self-esteem because . . . the kids would say, "How come he talks funny? How come he talks like a baby?" And so what happened is he stopped talking. And there would be days at preschool where he would go through the whole day without saying a word to a single person. And in preschool they were

having problems with him. He didn't want to talk and his self-esteem was low. He was easily intimidated. There was a long period of time when he would wet his pants every single day because he didn't want to ask the teacher to go to the bathroom. And we never knew it was hearing related until we had him screened for kindergarten. (Survey 186)

Difficulties with self-esteem were related not only to that child's different speech pattern in the years before the identification of his hearing loss but also to his use of hearing aids after identification.

Management of Hearing Aids

Despite the benefits of consistent amplification for hard of hearing children, hearing aid use is frequently less than optimal. Some parents believe that hearing aids are for use in school only. Others have a warranted concern about the safety and security of the hearing aids when used during play. For the survey, parents reported hearing aid use to be almost constant at school but more variable at home: At school 94% of HH children and 78% of DF children "always" wear their hearing aids, whereas 59% of HH children and 21% of DF children "always" wear their aids at home. The high cost of hearing aids and the fact that most insurance plans do not cover their costs make parents guard against damage or loss:

For awhile, everyone wanted to touch his hearing aids. I taught him to say, "You can't touch them, these cost $500 each! If anything happens, my mom will get very mad!" (Survey 186)

Another family lives in a small town and must travel many miles to receive needed services. This has made a difference in the kinds of support they have received and their satisfaction with services, including the provision of hearing aids. Suspecting their daughter's hearing loss when the child was 12 months old, the parents took her to a pediatrician, who delayed a hearing test for 6 months:

He made an appointment for us with an audiologist at [a university clinic many miles away]. We went and had the brain stem test, but she had an ear infection, so we went to an ENT [ear, nose, and throat specialist], and he put her on antibiotics, and then we went back and had her tested again. They went ahead and had her fitted with hearing aids. But they were real small hearing aids, and they weren't really powerful enough for her. So she had those for about 2 years, and then we went down to the [university clinic] again, and he put regular [brand name] hearing aids on her. And that really helped her speech a lot. . . . There just weren't a lot of services for parents who just found out. . . . There wasn't much of anything. . . . The audiologist wasn't that great, either. He seemed to be real overwhelmed [by her hearing loss], too. . . . He was a real young guy fresh out of school. I don't know whether he was just supersensitive or whether it just hurt him, too, but he seemed to be very overwhelmed by it himself. And he really didn't help much in the way of referrals or anything. (Survey 66)

The following mother of two hard of hearing daughters had a very different experience with audiologists and hearing aids:

Overall, for both of the girls, their audiologists were phenomenal. . . . They really have both offered me the most information. They talked a lot about etiology and prognosis, what I can expect, all of the nitty-gritty technical stuff about the hearing aids and exactly what they are hearing and even mentioning suggestions for future management. I think that both of them . . . have been the most helpful for me and also have given me the most information. (Survey 297)

The parents in the following excerpt chose "speech only" as their son's communication mode because of his successful use of hearing aids:

His hearing aids brought him within the outer edge of the average range in hearing. So his hearing was such that he could learn through that mode. He picked up speech sounds very well with therapy. So there wasn't a need to do anything different since he was very capable of learning that way. (Survey 242)

Hearing aids are one of the visible marks of hearing loss. Parents often have concerns that their children will be self-conscious about the aids or be teased about them by hearing classmates. The mother in the following selection explains how she promoted her son's acceptance of his hearing aids:

He's never been shy through any of this. Even when he first got his hearing aids, Kevin was never upset about them. We always used to joke about them in the beginning, "You want to hear Kevin beep?" You know, when kids would ask him what it is. But now everybody pretty much accepts everything because of the way we handled it. It's like, "Does your mother wear glasses?" "Well, Kevin wears hearing aids." That's how we dealt with it in the beginning, and he takes care of everything himself with those. (Survey 76)

Another child's response to his hearing aids was quite different. His mother believes that the reason is his late identification and the way the introduction of the aids was managed:

The ENT doctor told me, in front of my son, that he had to wear hearing aids. I said, "Hearing aids? How long?" And he said, "The rest of his life." I was stunned, and the doctor said, "Don't worry, he can keep his hair long so you can hide it." Hearing aids were something to be ashamed of. . . . And when we went to the preschool and explained to the teacher, her face fell and she said, "Oh, I'm so sorry!" Like he was dying or something. . . . So all along the way he got the message that [hearing aids are] not a good thing, and it's something wrong with him, and . . . he was very embarrassed with his hearing aids. (Survey 186)

That mother believes that her son's self-consciousness about his hearing aids contributed to his low self-esteem and that late identification made his adjustment more difficult.

Behavioral and Self-Esteem Concerns

The few studies that have focused on the social or behavioral status of hard of hearing children have reported severe problems for some children. One study of 40 children between 5 and 18 years of age with hearing losses of less than 61 dB showed that the parents rated their children as having "behavior problems that are characterized by aggression, impulsivity, immaturity, and resistance to discipline and structure" (Davis, Elfenbein, Schum, & Bentler, 1986, p. 60). Another study matched 25 children between 6 and 13 years of age with unilateral (in one ear only) hearing losses from 15 to 45 dB with 25 children without hearing losses. Scores on the Piers-Harris Children's Self-Concept Scale revealed no differences, but teachers rated the children, even with such minimal losses, more negatively "in the categories of dependence/independence, attention to task, emotional liability, and peer relations/social confidence" (Culbertson & Gilbert, 1986, p. 40). Finally, 33 students with unilateral hearing losses, ages 5 to 18, were evaluated with a brief screening instrument and found to be at risk for behavioral as well as academic difficulties (Dancer, Burl, & Waters, 1995).

Another research group compared 30 children with minimal sensorineural hearing losses (MSHL) to 105 hearing controls in grades 3, 6, and 9 on the teacher-completed Revised Behavior Problem Checklist. No significant differences between the two groups were found. However, a smaller group of MSHL children in grade 6 completed a self-report checklist and showed greater dysfunction than peers on "self-esteem" and "energy." Those in grade 9 showed greater dysfunction than peers for "social support," "stress," and "self-esteem" (Bess, Dodd-Murphy, & Parker, 1998).

Parents of children in the NPP survey identified 8% as having "behavior problems." Hard of hearing children were given significantly lower scores on the survey's behavior rating scale compared to deaf children (when those with additional conditions and those with deaf parents were excluded). Overall, however, the scores suggest that these parents do not see behavior as a serious problem. The consequences associated with behavioral concerns can be painful for the child and for family members, as the following illustrations show:

She has a younger brother and two younger sisters. She does have some rough times where she can be pretty mean, but I think that comes out of a lot of frustration. But other than that, we treat her just like the rest of them, and we don't make her hearing a priority as far as treating her differently because she can't hear. (Survey 211)

The child described in the first of the following excerpts came to live with her mother and stepfather when she was 3. Her hearing loss had not been identified, but she was enrolled in a special preschool for children with behavior problems:

When my wife and I first got married, her ex had custody [of their daughter]. And when we got her there were some behavioral problems, and that's why we put her [in that program], and then after she'd been in that program for about 6 months we found the hearing loss. We think that probably had something to do with the behavior problems, also. (Survey 85)

To me, of all the problems, self-esteem was the biggest. Because right now [at age 8] we've got over the speech problem. The only problem that lingers is the self-esteem. So that's a bigger problem than the hearing problem. . . . For us the damage was done when he was very young. (Survey 186)

Her biggest problem is her conduct, really. She has trouble paying attention for long periods of time and staying on task. (Survey 66)

Services Available to Parents

NPP survey data suggest that parents of hard of hearing children feel less well served than do parents of deaf children. Asked whether various services that early intervention programs often supply were available to them, parents of HH children replied "no" more frequently than parents of deaf children on six of seven items. These differences were significant for "information about deafness," "sign language instruction," and "parent groups." Differences were not significant for "information on legal rights," "information on behavior development," and "information on school choices." Fewer than half of either group had much access to "individual counseling": 36% of parents with deaf children and 45% of parents with hard of hearing children.

One mother of a hard of hearing child has written a book about her experiences: *Not Deaf Enough* (Candlish, 1996). She observes that professionals as well as parents too often take the position that deaf children need a great deal of extra help and attention but that hard of hearing children can manage very well if they are given hearing aids and preferential seating. Her son suffered from these attitudes. In addition, the parents of deaf children often avoided *her* because they believed that her child was more advantaged than theirs: "not deaf enough." That theme is echoed by one of the mothers we interviewed:

> *I went to the library to get books to help my son understand [his hearing loss]. And the only books that were available were for profoundly deaf people. There were several books about them but nothing related to him because he only has a high-frequency hearing loss. I was going to read him books and explain that it's not an unusual thing and talk through some of the fear. And books at that age are a wonderful means. I love books and raise my kids on books. So I always say, "When I retire I will try to write a book like that." (Survey 186)*

Hard of Hearing Children: Positive Coping

The previous interview excerpts from these parents of hard of hearing children omit or obscure important positive features that demonstrate the coping abilities of both children and parents. Examples occur in each and every interview of the parents' acceptance of their child's hearing status and of their attachment to and admiration for the child as a unique person with talents and endearing characteristics. These children are meeting and surpassing their parents' expectations:

> She's a wonderful, outgoing little girl. She's got lots of personality and a strong love for animals. . . . She's a wonderful kid, and I think deafness is part of her personality. She's got a terrific personality, she's very loving, she's a wonderful little kid. (Survey 24)

> She's very outgoing, on the go all the time. . . . She's always very bright, very seldom sad. . . . She's basically the light of my life. She's really coming along very well. (Survey 85)

> He's very active, he's typical, very well liked by his peers. . . . He's into sports and he has good skills. It's just his shyness or maybe lack of self-confidence holds him back, probably in several areas. Academically he's doing well. In math and probably PE. Just struggles a little in reading. (Survey 186)

> He's very energetic and active and a real good singer. He's got a wonderful personality, likes other kids, and he's a character. People really enjoy being around him. Loves . . . vehicles and anything he can take apart and explore, loves the outside. Very social. So he's a really delightful boy. (Survey 242)

> She's very outgoing, very outspoken. One of the things we've tried to stress with her, particularly since she's hearing impaired, is stress for her to be assertive. And she certainly is that. And she's very friendly. . . . She really lets people into her heart. (Survey 344)

Although paradoxical, it is sometimes the positive coping skills developed by hard of hearing children that contribute to their difficulties. They communicate very well in one-on-one and face-to-face interactions. Good speechreading skills may mask the extent of their hearing

difficulties, lulling parents and teachers into believing that they understand more than they actually do. Several studies of school-aged hard of
hearing children show that they have "far more educational and/or
communicative difficulty than was previously supposed" (Bess, 1985, p.
43). Comparisons of academic achievement of students with hearing
losses of 20 to 45 dB in grades 1 through 4 showed achievement scores
below those of controls in every grade (Blair, Peterson, & Viehweg,
1985). Children with unilateral hearing losses, ages 6 to 13, had lower
scores on academic tests and were more likely to have repeated a grade
compared to hearing controls (Culbertson & Gilbert, 1986). These children will need special services throughout their school years if their
achievements are to match their intellectual abilities.

Conclusion

Hard of hearing children and their families need more services that
address the specific problems related to minimal hearing losses. Professionals, as well as parents, often assume that once these children are fitted with hearing aids, they will function like children without a hearing
loss. Long-delayed identification and intervention create many negative
consequences. These include delays in language learning for children and
self-blame or guilt for parents. Parent support groups or counseling
opportunities specifically for parents of hard of hearing children could
help to alleviate some of these secondary effects.

Future cohorts of children with minimal hearing loss should benefit
from the growing practice of universal newborn hearing screening. In
some areas where this has been introduced, the average age of identification of hearing loss has already been reduced to 6 months (Yoshinaga-
Itano, Sedey, Coulter, & Mehl, 1998). Three years after the study by
Yoshinaga-Itano et al., identification in Colorado was reported to occur
on average between 2 and 3 months of age, reflecting the rapidity of
change in this arena (Yoshinaga-Itano & Marion Downs Center for Infant
Hearing, 2001). However, newborn screening will not obviate the need
for continued screening during the preschool years, particularly if we are

to be able to identify children whose minimal hearing losses stem from repeated ear infections, illnesses, or accidents.

Despite many advances in procedures of identification and intervention, hard of hearing children continue to be forgotten and overlooked in comparison to children with severe and profound hearing losses. To be "not deaf enough" subjects children and their parents to unnecessary disadvantages.

Chapter 4
Additional Conditions: It Takes a Team

With her other disabilities . . . you know, I had more than just the hearing to think about. She had a lot of surgeries and stuff. (Survey 149)

He's a walking, breathing miracle. (Survey 16)

Providing services to children with a hearing loss and conditions such as developmental delays, blindness, cerebral palsy, or behavioral problems challenges professionals who serve this population (Giangreco, Edelman, MacFarland, & Luiselli, 1997; Jones & Jones, in press; Powers, Elliott, Patterson, Shaw, & Taylor, 1995). Nationwide, about 40% of children with a hearing loss have an additional disability according to the 1999–2000 Annual Survey of Deaf and Hard of Hearing Children and Youth (Gallaudet Research Institute, 2001). This chapter focuses on the experiences of parents with deaf or hard of hearing children who have a visual, cognitive, or physical disability or a behavioral problem that might affect their development or education.

Mothers whose babies have both a hearing loss and another condition report patterns of stress that are different from those of mothers whose children have a hearing loss only (Meadow-Orlans, Smith-Gray, & Dyssegaard, 1995). Parenting stress scores for mothers whose children are deaf or hard of hearing and have another condition tended to be either extremely high (reflecting great stress) or extremely low (reflecting denial of stress). Thus, the experiences of these families suggest variations in ability to cope and a greater need for support compared to other families. In a study of German parents, Hintermair (2000a) found that parents of children who are deaf or hard of hearing and have an additional condition experience increased stress because of their complex situation. The stress becomes more intense when the children have behavior problems and need more attention from their caregivers.

Participant Characteristics

In the NPP survey 32% of the respondents reported that their child had one or more disabilities or behavioral problems that might affect their development or education. The percentages by type of disability are reported from three sources in Table 4-1: the Annual Survey of Deaf and Hard of Hearing Children and Youth for 1996–1997 (Holden-Pitt & Diaz, 1998), the NPP, and the subgroup who participated in the telephone and focus group interviews. The interviewed sample included children with the full spectrum of disabilities, including those who have a visual impairment, a learning disability, a developmental delay, an attention deficit, a behavior problem, cerebral palsy, or some other condition. About 70% of the 23 interviewed parents reported that their child had more than one condition in addition to the hearing loss.

Seventeen of the 23 children with additional conditions were boys (74%). Ten of the mothers (43%) were African American or Hispanic or were in mixed-race marriages. Eleven of the children (48%) were hard of hearing, while the remainder were deaf.

The following descriptions give a picture of the children this chapter discusses:

His name is David. He is 8 years old, and he has cerebral palsy on his left side, and he is hearing impaired. It is profound in his right ear and moderate to profound in his left. So he wears two hearing aids, and he does sign and he reads lips, and he's learning how to read. And that's about it. Ya know, he's a sweet little boy. He has asthma, and he's on medication for seizures. Other than that he's just like a normal little kid, and you would never be able to tell he has all these problems. (Survey 334)

He's Anthony. He's not like any kid I've even been around before. And part of that is he was born with some extra challenges. And so he's been slow with his motor delays. He's very outgoing though, very friendly, very boisterous, and all boy. (Survey 257)

Table 4-1. Proportions of Children with Conditions in Addition to Hearing Loss

Source			
Type of condition	Annual Survey of Deaf and Hard of Hearing Children and Youth 1996–1997 (Holden-Pitt & Diaz, 1998)[a]	NPP[b]	Interviews and Focus Groups Cited in This Chapter[c]
No additional condition	66%	68%	0%
Vision impairment	4	8	30
Learning disability	9	5	9
Mental retardation/ developmental delay	8	12	30
Attention deficit disorder	Not reported	9	26
Serious emotional disturbance/behavior problem	4	9	13
Cerebral palsy/ orthopedic condition	Not reported	6	43
Other conditions[d]	Not reported	29	48
Total children (frequency)	31,760	393	23

a. The Annual Survey data are not actually comparable with either the NPP or the interview/focus group data in that the survey results include only four categories of disabilities and do not indicate how children with multiple disabilities were included. Moreover, the numbers do not add up to 100%; the authors, however, do not explain why.

b. In the NPP responses, respondents could check more than one type of additional condition. The data are based on the total number of conditions checked, and therefore the percentages do not total 100%.

c. The parents for this chapter were selected specifically because their children had conditions in addition to hearing loss. Thus, the row for "no additional condition" for this group is zero. The respondents could indicate more than one type of condition. The data are based on the total number of conditions checked, and therefore the percentages do not total 100%.

d. Includes brain damage, epilepsy, and other health conditions.

Themes Based on Parents' Responses

The parents of children with additional disabilities offered many helpful thoughts. The themes that emerged include parents' descriptions of their children and parenting experiences, circumstances surrounding identification of hearing loss, challenges, early services provided or needed, behavior problems that complicate the delivery of services, and satisfaction with services. We use these themes to organize the remainder of this chapter.

Parenting Experiences: Struggles and Successes

These parents described their early experiences in a way that is qualitatively different from that of the parents of children without additional conditions. The nature of the condition influenced parents' descriptions of their experiences. Some parents whose children had physical disabilities had frequent interactions with the medical community. Two mothers described their fears in these situations:

> *[H]e's always been in the hospital since he was born. In and out, in and out. At the time, I thought that he's not going to make it. Always in the hospital and I was always crying, and I was like "My God, what happened?"* (Focus Group 2)

> *A lot of times when you have a child that is very ill or has an uncertain future, the medical profession is hesitant to just tell you what they're thinking. And so you end up worrying about things you don't even have to worry about because no one will say, "I think this is happening," or "I think that's happening."* (Survey 121)

Other parents described their experiences as exceedingly stressful. One mother said if she had known about all of the problems that she would have, she would not have had additional children. Another described taking antidepressant medications to deal with stress.

Several parents recognized the mixed feelings of sadness and inspiration that they felt. When the children survived life-threatening episodes, they celebrated their child as a wonderful human being who happened to have a permanent disability. From these children they derived pride and strength that helped them adjust:

> *And when I'm feeling, you know, kind of lonely or sad or think that there are so many problems in this world and why? Why me? I just look at my son and his hope. He's a miracle and he's loved.* (Focus Group 2)

> *As to my experience, oh God—I would not ever trade Chris. I would not have missed having Chris, because until he came, experiencing life (pause)—ordinary life. This kid is thrilled with animals, with birds. It's the most awesome thing. It's like God himself, Jesus, has given him such a gift for noticing all the different animals. And it really reminds you of a simpler time maybe, and you learn to respect what really is important and to appreciate more. Much more.* (Survey 16)

> *I'm proud of him because he depends on himself. He has cerebral palsy and he don't walk. He tries to walk and he do everything on his own. But what hurts, it hurts a little bit because every time I try to help him, he tell me NO, he do it on his own. And I'm proud of him for that, but I like to be with him. But he don't like that. And I thought it would be a little hard for him even though he don't walk, but it don't bother him. It used to bother me, but it don't bother me no more because I see that it don't bother him, so it don't bother me. And I'm proud of him.* (Focus Group 2)

Identification: Sometimes Aided by Additional Conditions, Sometimes Masked

Identification of hearing loss for children with additional disabilities tends to occur later than for children without such conditions. In the NPP survey, children without additional conditions were identified at age 21.7 months; those with additional conditions were identified at 23.0 months.

(Even though the average ages are quite similar, the difference is statistically significant because the spread and variation were larger for the group with additional conditions than for others.) These data support the idea that the presence of another condition may at times mask the presence of, and thus allay suspicions of, a hearing loss. For some families this was the case, but for others, the additional condition provided an early warning that alerted medical professionals to suggest a hearing test. The following excerpts describe some situations in which an additional condition contributed to an early diagnosis:

> *Because of that she had other problems. I mean she has microcephaly, she had gross motor delays, and so [the doctor] thought as long as she's there, why don't we have her hearing checked?* (Survey 75)

> *My son was working on a lot of problems, too. He was in the hospital for 5 weeks. . . . The problems he had could cause him to be deaf. So they tested him before he left the hospital, so I knew when he was 5 weeks old that he was deaf. But I was just so happy he was alive.* (Focus Group 2)

> *When we came here to America, I came here about, with him, 5 years ago. And they did a surgery here, open-heart surgery, and they said, "Didn't you know that your son is deaf?" and I said, "Oh, it could have been worse."* (Focus Group 2)

In at least two families, language delay was attributed to the presence of an additional disability, so concerns about hearing loss were not raised initially:

> *I heard the doctor say that, you know, she was born with a cleft palate and stuff like that. So they always said, well, she would be a little delayed talking. So we just, I assumed, you know, she wasn't talking that good, it was due to the cleft palate. And then, you know, whenever we'd take her in, you know, 'cuz once a year they have the cleft palate clinics, and there was always some, I guess, concern about her hearing, but they could never*

really get a good hearing test. And finally the one, you know, said, well, let's try, and they got a good one, and yeah, she has a good hearing loss. (Survey 306)

Then he still wasn't talking at the same time, so right after he turned 3 the doctor said, "Ya know, he's still not talking. I understand you may think it has to do with the cerebral palsy, but let's just check his hearing to rule that out." And they did an ABR test, and we found that he's hearing impaired. That's why he wasn't talking. . . . We thought he wasn't talking because of the cerebral palsy. It was really strong on one side, and we thought maybe it affected his speech, too. And that wasn't the reason. The reason why he wasn't speaking was because he was hearing impaired. (Survey 334)

Jones and Jones (in press) report that hearing loss can mask other disabilities as well. The challenge is to differentiate between language delays that are related to communication access and those related to other disabilities. The situation is complicated because disabilities such as autism and other pervasive developmental disorders often include significant language delays.

Reaction to Diagnosis
Parents have a wide range of reactions to multiple disabilities:

At the 3-months' visit they tested him for the hearing and the vision. And the doctor told us at that visit that he was deaf and blind and mentally retarded. And I can't remember which caught me by surprise the most. But, um, I think I expected the hearing loss. But the vision, I don't think I expected. (Survey 73)

When we found out he had cerebral palsy, OK, that hit us like a ton of bricks, but we had a chance to deal with that. OK, we'll get over that. We'll get through that, no big deal. Then we found out he was hearing impaired, ya know, and they just tell you. When you go in the office, they just tell you, "Well, your kid is this and he's that and he can't hear this and he can't hear [that] and . . . " [they] just blurt it all out to ya. So we walked out of that office feelin' like we had been knocked in the chest. And we got over that. We said, "OK, we can deal with that. No big deal. He can get hearing aids; we'll learn sign language, all that stuff." And then he had the seizures, and ya know it—everything didn't happen all at once. So it gave us a chance to, ya know, get through one thing at a time. (Survey 334)

And we had, by the time they did the test on his hearing, they had ruled out some genetic anomalies that they thought were fatal and—and decided that this was just a series of birth defects, so the hearing loss was not the most important thing on our list. It was sorta minor compared to everything else. We were grateful that he was going to come home and grow up. So we figured, you know, we'd deal with that. So it didn't come as quite the shock it would have, had he not had all these other problems. (Survey 121)

One child's hearing loss had been identified, but the doctor would not believe that she was having seizures:

She was having seizures for 4 months, and the neurologist would not believe me. They did an EEG and the EEG was normal. He wouldn't believe me. Since then I've found out that quite often EEGs can be normal for kids with epilepsy. It just might not be picking up. The seizures might be so deep that it's just not picking up on it. So I mean a positive EEG can just sort of confirm it and can sort of tell you what location of the brain. But just because the EEG is normal doesn't rule out epilepsy. He wouldn't believe me that she was having seizures—partial seizures—at the time. She didn't start having the full grand mal seizures. It wasn't until several months later we were at the doctor's—my pediatrician's—office for something totally different, and she had a seizure in front of my pediatrician. (Survey 75)

For some children, an accurate diagnosis continues to be a problem. One child was developmentally delayed, had poor speech, and was deaf. He was being evaluated to determine whether he was autistic:

> *He gets focused on one thing, and they're trying to see if he can be tested for autism to see if that's what is causing the singleness. . . . He's usually not aware of, you know, like if somebody's teaching him. He's not aware of that. He's being harassed; he just thinks they are playing with him. He really likes things, like he'll decide that he likes owls, and then every single thing has to be owls. You know he carries the owls around, he'll draw pictures of owls, everything is owls. And then it changed to Pinocchio when Pinocchio came out. Just one thing, you know, at a time. He can't seem to do more than one thing, focus on more than one thing.* (Survey 115)

Challenges: Understanding the Meaning of a Disability

A child with an additional condition increases the cognitive demands parents encounter. They have to learn not only about hearing loss and its complexities but also about other disabling conditions. One mother did not understand the meaning of cerebral palsy and asked the doctors to explain it. Another mother was told, "Your child has cytomegalovirus"— a term that was foreign to her:

> *At the time, it would [have] been nice if the doctors would've sat down and explained it more instead of just little bits and pieces, making comments when we would go. And then expecting me to go look up things on my own. . . . I mean they may be very busy, and they may have their appointments all backed up, but I told the one teacher this before: I didn't know about the cytomegalovirus. It would've been nice . . . if they'd have had some research or helpful information on it right there for us to read it. Instead of me having to go out when I got home and hunt it out on my own, 'cuz I didn't know where to go.* (Survey 16)

Giangreco, Cloninger, Mueller, Yuan, and Ashworth (1991) report that parents of children with multiple disabilities expressed fears about knowing what to do and whether they could handle the challenges of their children's conditions. For example, one mother was afraid that her disturbed son would hurt his siblings. For another mother, seizures complicated the life of her child:

They had a developmental specialist working with her for about 8 months. When the seizures were really severe, and I mean, because she was losing so much developmentally and she was just having so many seizures and was basically like in and out of the hospital and doctor's appointments that they started becoming concerned that she was going to start losing ground developmentally. (Survey 75)

Services: Multiple Conditions, Multiple Needs

Children with multiple conditions need a range of services, and parents appreciated professionals who saw their child as a child first (Giangreco et al., 1991). One mother described hospital nurses who cared for her newborn with multiple problems:

Right after he was born, we were told that he had this genetic problem and that he would live a short and painful life . . . and the nurses treated him differently. They treated him like a baby, even though he had all these problems. They treated him like a human being, and that was very meaningful for us. (Survey 121)

Some children benefited because an additional condition was the basis for extra home visits specific to their special needs. One mother described her child's earliest program:

It's a program for developing, you know, for special needs kids. When they are babies, they will come out to the home and work with the child and stuff like that until they are 3. Once they are 3, then they can go on to, like I say, this preschool for special needs kids. (Survey 306)

Another child had the advantage of a program addressing both his hearing loss and his physical disability:

You know they had like a table with sand in it. And they say that children with CP, they lose like their sense of touch. They don't have a strong sense, they can't feel different textures. You know, their arms and hands aren't as sensitive. So they would let him put his hands in the sand and let him feel the different types of dry sand and damp sand and wet sand, rice, and beans and let him run his fingers through it. They would have swimming parties and let him feel how cold the water feels. Let him feel how bumble balls feel, beach balls are, let them feel how the air feels when it's in it, let them feel how the air feels when it's out of it. They go around the circle and ask them. They count every day, the calendar. They would just learn little different things. They had like circle time, and they would sing their good-morning songs in sign language whether the kids were hearing impaired or not in that class. He just learned so much. (Survey 334)

However, finding appropriate services was a challenge for some parents. The mother of a daughter with microcephaly reported an unsatisfactory visit to a pediatric neurologist who said:

"Oh, my God, she has all these problems . . . and you'll need all these services, and she should be in an early intervention program, getting physical therapy." And I said, "Well, where do I find that?" And . . . his remark was, "I don't know. It'll probably be really hard, you know, you probably won't be able to, but that's what she needs." (Survey 75)

The doctor gave her no referrals. After much effort she found services appropriate for her child's needs. Some participants got information from mothers whose children had similar problems or from a library.

Support groups for such parents increase both the size of the social support network and the perceived helpfulness of peers (Krauss, Upshur, Shonkoff, & Hauser-Cram, 1993). Parent support groups can improve participants' ability to cope with their child's problems (Singer et al., 1999).

Inappropriate Services

An audiologist used a child's cerebral palsy as an excuse to withhold hearing aids and sign language instruction because "Well, there are some social ramifications to wearing a hearing aid, and he has enough hearing in one of his ears so he functions" (Survey 121). Based on this recommendation, the parents did not get hearing aids. Later, when their son was in a preschool for children with cerebral palsy, he was reassessed. Another audiologist prescribed an aid that was placed in the wrong ear. Finally he was enrolled in a school for deaf and blind children:

> And it wasn't until he got into kindergarten, when he got to our regional school for the deaf and blind, that the audiologist there said, "The hearing in his bad ear is so distorted that if you amplify it, it's just amplifying distortion. So put the hearing aid in his good ear, and it will get it to almost normal hearing." And we saw a big improvement when we started doing that. And we kinda screwed up for the first 5 years as far as finding out how to fine-tune his amplification. (Survey 121)

One adaptive physical education teacher prescribed activities that were inappropriate for a child with physical limitations. The mother described how the teacher evaluated the children:

> "Throw with your right arm, throw it with your left arm, throw it overhead with your right arm, throw it overhead with your left arm, and throw it overhead with both arms." And he couldn't do some of those things because he's got a left-sided weakness. He can't throw it with both. He can't take it with both arms extended all the way. He just, those are things he can't do, and they just mark him down on that. But we had to go and have a talk with her and say, "Look, I know, I understand you're

doing your job, but don't give him a hard time if he can't do it. He just—
it is medically, it's physically impossible for him. Don't give him a hard time
because it frustrates him even more, and then he doesn't want to do it at
all. And then the things he can do, he doesn't want to do because he's frus-
trated." He's really a good child though. He's very good. (Survey 334)

Another mother indicated that her daughter was not allowed to attend
a program for deaf children because of her developmental delays:

She goes to a regular elementary school, but she's in a handicapped class,
multiple handicapped class, and . . . we have inquired about the deaf
school here, but they won't take her because of her developmental prob-
lems. (Survey 368)

Another concern arose because of the diverse needs that professionals
must address in a classroom for children with additional disabilities. One
mother explained:

They need to be better staffed or because there's just, you know, like I say,
it's been so mixed in, you got a deaf child with blind kids and other hand-
icapped kids and you know, don't misunderstand me, I'm not putting the
kids down. It's just that these kids are not getting, you know, enough on
their level of what they need in that school day because this teacher's hav-
ing to teach two or three different things in that classroom. (Survey 118)

The severity of some children's disabilities requires the use of adaptive
technologies:

Well, they use pictures and symbols at school. And they put the picture
symbols on the switch, and that's one thing that I know of. And they try

picture symbols with tactile surfaces. That's a good idea. And it's got four little buttons, like 2 inches in diameter. And you can record whatever you want, and it can be four different messages, like "I want to eat," "I want my toys," "I want music." . . . And he pushes the button. And he's got that. . . . I don't even like to use it because it's like not challenging at all. I think he can do more. I want him to say it. I mean he says "Mom." He's been saying "Mom" forever. So my theory is if he can say "Mom," he can say other things. (Survey 73)

This mother feared that the professionals' low expectations unnecessarily limited her son to the communication board. Awareness of such concerns can lead to improved relationships between parents and professionals and to more effective communication for children as well.

Behavior Challenges and Services

Children with behavior problems present special challenges to their parents, other family members, and professionals. Elsewhere researchers have suggested that frustration with communication may result in behavioral problems (Mertens, Sass-Lehrer, & Scott-Olson, 2000; Pipp-Siegel, Sedey, & Yoshinaga-Itana, 2002). One mother believed that her child's behavior problems resulted from early communicative frustrations:

I just believe that, I don't know if, I could be sounding ridiculous to you . . . that is when they really need to learn. And I just think missing out on all that and how he used to behave. I mean we couldn't go anywhere. We couldn't have people over and if we did it was horrible. (Survey 31)

This appeared to be the case for several of the parents. However, this mother acknowledged that she might have contributed to the behavior problems by being too permissive:

I overprotect him and I do all the bad things that moms do, ya know. Let
him get away with this and that and the other thing. So I've helped on this
behavior business. (Survey 31)

Another family adopted a boy with serious behavioral problems. They
thought the behavior problems were not related entirely to deafness but
also to early abusive experiences. The dad said:

Behaviorally, we have some problems, but we don't attribute that to the
deafness, we attribute it to the neglectful environment that he was in for
those few years. He does come . . . from a real negative history, a lot of
neglect and quite possibly abuse. There have been some behavioral issues
and acting out, but this is not all—maybe the deafness comes in only
because he didn't fully understand what was going on in his environment.
He didn't learn language, pick it up and hear what was going on. Maybe
that had some negative effects, but we are dealing with some behavioral
issues now. (Survey 218)

In chapter 3 a parent described punishing her daughter for misbehav-
ior before she knew about the child's hearing loss. That parent received
help from the school and her family in dealing with the behavior problems. Some parents felt that schools exerted too much behavior control;
others felt they were too lenient:

The teacher he has right now is very structured, and she's, you know, "You
sit in your seats and you do this and you do this." And he can't sit for long
periods of time, and he gets real distracted. . . . I'm not saying it's good or
bad. I'm just saying for him personally it's hard because he doesn't sit, you
know? He doesn't sit and color; he doesn't sit and watch TV. He doesn't
do things like that. And I don't know if it's that he gets bored or he's just
—you know, because he is delayed, he can't follow everything that's being
said, you know. I just don't know why he's having such a struggle in the

classroom. But I know noises bother him really bad, and if there's a lot of noise or something, he'll get to shaking and he can't deal with a lot of noise. (Survey 115)

He's just very hyperactive. . . . He's doing pretty good in school. He just has the problem of being attentive to something a certain amount of time. He tends to want to ramble around, BUT, nothing against my school. They just—they let him get by with a little too much, ya know? They don't want to say, "Hey, you're gonna do it," and he knows who he can fool and who he can't. (Survey 118)

And it seems that teachers let them get away with stuff that they don't let nonhandicapped students get away with. And that always bothers me. I don't know why the teachers allow that. If it's just easier or what. That's my opinion. And it really bothers me that I can go in the classroom, and he'll be in the back of the classroom playing Legos, and none of the other kids are allowed to. And she'll say, "Well, he just got tired of doing his work." (Survey 115)

I feel like that they should make the kids work more, you know, in the sense of curriculum, academic work, because I don't see that they're being like, you take 'em out and put 'em beside another school. They're not working on what this [hearing] school would have worked on all day. I just don't feel like they're being taught like they should. (Survey 118)

In addition to the concerns related to low expectations for their children, parents also expressed concerns about safety. In one school a child was able to leave the classroom and wander out onto the playground or off of the school grounds:

Now this year, they've had a problem a couple of times, because he will get permission to go to the bathroom and then they'll find him outside playing. . . . They lost him twice at the child development center because he just walked off, you know, he just wandered off. Even though there was an aide out there watching. He was just such a quiet, nonaggressive little boy that he just wandered off, and nobody would realize it. Like when he left the classroom those two times, the police couldn't help him because he couldn't talk and communicate enough for them to figure out who he was and where he'd come from. (Survey 115)

In some cases children did not receive needed services because the school staff could not control their behavior:

I was happy with the teacher, but I wasn't happy with the speech therapist's antics . . . because they weren't giving him what he was supposed to have on his IEP [Individualized Educational Plan], because they couldn't control him. . . . The one deaf child in the school and he wasn't getting speech therapy. (Survey 286)

He was supposed to be transitioning into the regular classroom, but the teacher couldn't deal with him. And she finally just gave up and said she couldn't deal with him. That he was too disruptive to the class and that he would just get up and walk out of the classroom and stuff. And she couldn't keep an eye on him. (Survey 115)

He didn't speak at all. He would always be crying. He was in Head Start, and they had to take him out of Head Start because he didn't want to go. It was real terrible. (Focus Group 2)

Parents also described the importance of good communication with the school. One parent complained:

I would say that the teachers need to be more informative to the parents. I mean there's a lot of times that there will be an incident where he and one of the other kids would, you know, not really fight, just you know how boys will be boys. And then I get an incident report like 2 weeks later . . . and I'm at the school every day, every morning and every afternoon. And

I'm not told any of this. And then I'm getting these incident letters saying that this happened, or this happened on such and such a day, but they didn't tell me and I was there. (Survey 118)

Positive Experiences: Satisfaction with Effective Services

Some schools, however, did have an effective method for communicating with the family about behavioral problems:

We're so thrilled because they're willing to keep the parents so closely involved in dealing with his behavior problems. This is a . . . boy who's been suspended three times just this last year. So we have some behavior problems in the school. You know, we sit down and we have meetings and we're included and they're actually saying, "Well, what works at home? Do you think this would work? Have you tried this?" And we would request daily contact with the teachers, and they give us daily contact. (Survey 218)

Parents who had access to a counselor who could sign expressed appreciation for that ability. One father who had adopted a boy with a history of early abuse felt it was important to have a signing counselor:

He sees a counselor at the local mental health agency. He sees her every 3 weeks. This we began because of some of the acting-out behaviors. Just to have somebody to talk to—to explore. He's been kicked out of school a few times because of angry outbursts and tantrums and also because we thought we're seeing these behaviors in school and it might be related to what happened 4 or 5 years ago. Although he doesn't talk a lot about 4 or 5 years ago, it'd be nice to get a professional involved now and then as he moves into his teenage years. If he becomes a real problem, at least we've laid the ground rules down. . . . It took us a long time to search out the counselor that we have now. We were a little bit disappointed that we

don't have more fluent ASL or any form of sign in professionals in the
counseling area. (Survey 218)

This last comment illustrates that having access to counselors who can communicate directly with the children becomes more important as the children become older.

Conclusions

The stress felt by the parents cited in this chapter highlights the need to understand the real challenges in the everyday lives of these families and to provide the information and support they need. Parents celebrate the miracle of their child's survival and achievements while acknowledging the stress that the challenges create. Parents know there is much to learn with a child who is deaf or hard of hearing—and still more to learn with an additional disabling condition. A child's diverse needs can complicate the obtaining of appropriate services. For example, if behavior problems are greater than those a program is prepared to manage, services may be withheld, despite their importance.

Powers et al. (1995) report finding more stress among families where deaf or hard of hearing children had additional conditions than among families with deaf or hard of hearing children without additional conditions. Professionals and parents agreed that maladaptive behaviors interfered with the child's social and emotional readiness to learn. Many teachers and parents are not prepared to meet the needs of students with multiple conditions, especially of those from families under a great deal of stress. A team approach is necessary for successful intervention with children with multiple disabilities, and the provision of support services that reduce parental stress should be a top priority. Teachers, psychologists, and counselors are critical members of such teams.

One avenue might be to have parents who are in the same situation share experiences (Hintermair, 2000b). This can help both in identifying needed services and in providing parental networks for social support. Special support networks are available for parents who have a physical or sensory disability themselves (Meadow–Orlans, 2002a). Medical professionals could be made aware of these resources so that they could recommend the additional avenues of support for parents of deaf and hard of hearing children with additional conditions.

A number of issues that arose in the study of this subgroup suggest opportunities for future research. For example, researchers could investigate trends in the identification of various conditions in children. If the children in this study were followed over time, would the incidence of the various conditions change? And if so, how? Many resources that provide models for services are presented in Appendix D. Research could reveal the strengths and weaknesses of these models, as well as provide guidance in applying them in different contexts.

Chapter 5

Deaf and Hard of Hearing Parents: High Expectations

She was a child first. I didn't want to treat her any differently just because she's deaf. I wanted my expectations to be high for her. I didn't want to think, "Oh, she can't do this because she's deaf." I wanted her to have a fair chance. (Survey 260)

The situations of deaf parents and of their deaf children have improved greatly in the past several decades. Parents' expectations for their children are higher, they demand more from their children's schools, and the legal system and the general public view them as competent to rear either birth children or adoptive children.

This has not always been the case. As recently as 1967 a California judge ruled that a couple—simply because they were deaf—should not be permitted to adopt a child. This decision was reversed on appeal on the grounds that the adoptive parents' right to due process and equal protection of the law had been violated (Gilhool & Gran, 1985; Meadow-Orlans, 2002a). In a 1985 case a Michigan court awarded custody of the hearing children of a deaf mother to grandparents, believing that the children needed daily exposure to speech. This decision, too, was overturned by an appeals court (Geer, 1985). In contrast, a father who was interviewed for this study described the relative ease with which he and his deaf wife adopted a 5-month-old Korean baby:

In Korea they did not know she was deaf. The parents from [a Midwestern state] adopted her. . . . They found her deaf so they did not want her. So the agency found our name [and] called us if we would like to adopt her. . . . We [had previously] applied [for an] adoption and waited for 2 years. So we almost gave up the adoption process. Somehow

the agency called us, they found a girl. We said, "Wow!" We expected we
would get her in a month or so. They said, "No, you get her next day." We
were in shock. We were not ready, and we did not even have any baby
stuff. (Survey 177)

The readiness of the agency to process the deaf couple's application reflects changes in the legal system that support the rights of deaf parents.

Other factors have also contributed to society's views of deaf parents' capabilities (Meadow-Orlans, 2002b). Several studies conducted in the 1960s and 1970s show that deaf children with deaf parents performed at higher academic levels and were better adjusted socially than deaf children with hearing parents (Brasel & Quigley, 1977; Meadow, 1968; Stuckless & Birch, 1966; Vernon & Koh, 1970). Later studies found that deaf preschool children with deaf parents differed from hearing peers neither in social behavior nor in attachment patterns (Meadow, Greenberg, Erting, & Carmichael, 1981; Meadow, Greenberg, & Erting, 1985). Recent research on interactions of mother-child dyads shows deaf mothers to be highly responsive to their deaf infants and preschool children (Jamison, 1994; Meadow-Orlans, 1997; Spencer, 2000a). They modify signed communication to maximize infants' visual input and increase tactile contact that helps to replace infants' reduced auditory contact with the environment (Erting, Prezioso, & Hynes, 1994; Erting, Thumann-Prezioso, & Benedict, 2000; Mohay, 2000). Thus, research reinforces the idea that deaf people are not only capable of providing supportive environments for their deaf children but may in many ways be better prepared than hearing parents (Meadow-Orlans, 2002a).

Deaf NPP Participants and Their Children

The 34 deaf and hard of hearing mothers responding to the NPP survey were more likely to identify their children as "deaf" rather than "hard of hearing" compared to hearing mothers (67% versus 44%). Children with deaf parents were less likely to have additional conditions, compared to those with hearing parents (18% versus 32%).

Ten deaf or hard of hearing parents participated in follow-up telephone interviews: Two hard of hearing mothers responded to spoken questions; five deaf mothers and one deaf father responded by TTY; and two deaf mothers responded through a hearing interpreter. The 10 interviewees were representative of parents and children in the survey: Children were evenly divided between boys and girls; two were hard of hearing, eight were deaf, and one had an additional condition. Parents in one family were African American, one parent was of mixed race, and eight were White; all of the parents used sign language (seven used ASL at home, and three used English plus ASL or PSE). Themes emerging from these interviews included response to the identification of hearing loss; attitudes about hearing aids and speech training; educational and social concerns; and level of satisfaction with early services.

Response to Identification of Hearing Loss

For the 25 survey children with two deaf parents, hearing loss was suspected at an average age of 4 months and confirmed at an average age of 9 months. Among the 295 survey children with two hearing parents, hearing loss was suspected at an average age of 17 months and confirmed at 22 months. These dramatic differences might be predicted since many deaf parents anticipate the birth of a deaf child because of the known genetic component in their own hearing loss. This expectation of identification and familiarity with deafness leads most deaf parents to a quick acceptance of the condition:

I'm the third generation of a deaf family, and having a deaf child was kind of expected. (Survey 27)

Interviewer: When he was diagnosed, did you have any concerns?

Parent: Not really, because deafness runs in my family. I have deaf grandparents, parents, [and] many [other deaf] relatives. (Survey 209)

When Polly was born, I knew immediately that she was deaf, too. It is hereditary. . . . Both [children] were diagnosed by audiologist at hospital . . . at birth. (Survey 313)

However, not all deaf parents *expect* a child to be deaf:

When we were told he was deaf, we were not disappointed because we are deaf, too. We were just shocked because we do not have any deaf in our family for generations. So we were thrilled. (Survey 316)

There are many complexities, and no family reaction can be predicted. This is powerfully illustrated by a hard of hearing mother who is married to a deaf man. She described her feelings about the identification of hearing status for each of her four children:

If I had a deaf child and I never knew any deaf people or never learned sign language growing up, I would be devastated. But my attitude [would be] that I'd be so thankful that that was the only thing they had wrong with them. I was just so thankful when [our first child] was diagnosed as deaf. I was just relieved that that's all she was. And then, of course, I wasn't real surprised when [our second child] was diagnosed deaf. I didn't even have her tested until she was several months old because I already knew it. And then when [the third child] was diagnosed hearing, it was, like, a shock. And my husband accused me of being upset. I said, "No, I'm not upset. I'm just so shocked." Yet it's been so exciting for me because it's so nice to have somebody to talk to and talk back to me, you know. Then when [the fourth child] was diagnosed deaf, I was really sad. You know, I mean I had these four healthy children, and I was so thrilled with that. . . . They have all their fingers and toes, they seem to be very bright . . . but when [baby number four] came along as deaf I was really sad. I wanted [my hearing child] to have a buddy, somebody that he could talk to. Hmmm, not that he can't. . . . I know I was really close to my hard of hearing brother because I could talk to him and he'd talk to me. Even though we were 10 years apart, I was always closer to him than I was close to the others. Until, of course, we all became adults. . . . It was just a strange kind of emotion. I was sad and I knew [she was deaf] before they tested her, but . . . I didn't realize that she would be so deaf that she wouldn't register anything. It was just sad. I can imagine that's what so many hearing parents [feel]. (Survey 260)

Another mother reported her observations of factors that create differences in the responses of deaf people to infants' hearing status:

[I] often think when deaf parents have deaf children they feel closer to them, and I know some of them [are] going to be happy when they have [a] deaf infant. It really varies on who and what kind of people. What kind of society they come from. If you [go to a] mainstream school . . . they'd rather to have hearing baby. I'm not biased, but I think it's how things are now. (Survey 209)

As the status of deaf people has improved over the last several decades (Meadow-Orlans, 2001), attitudes of deaf people regarding deaf children have changed. One researcher who conducted many interviews with hearing adult children of deaf parents reported that his informants commented on the increasing number of younger deaf adults who wanted deaf children. "The stigma of having a 'defective' child was increasingly displaced by wanting to have a child who was like themselves" (Preston, 1994, p. 192). The reminiscence of a deaf woman who grew up in a deaf family illustrates this change over time:

My parents were rather disappointed that both of their children were deaf. They felt this way because at that time deafness was viewed as pathological. My parents were actually pressured by my father's parents (who were themselves deaf) not to bear any more children! My paternal grandmother, who was deaf, became pregnant after having my father. Her family members who were hearing weren't too happy about the possibility of her bearing another deaf child. This influenced her to choose to have an abortion. What made matters worse, she discovered that she had aborted a set of twins! Nowadays many Deaf parents *want* deaf children, but in those days it was different. (Searls & Johnston, 1996, pp. 204–205)

Hearing Aids and Speech Training

Deaf parents may not immediately seek speech training or acquire hearing aids for their deaf and hard of hearing children (Meadow-Orlans & Sass-Lehrer, 1995). Deaf participants in the NPP survey reported an average lag between identification of hearing loss and hearing aid acquisition of 19 months and a lag of 14 months for initiation of speech training. Comparable lags for children with hearing parents were 7 months and 9 months, respectively. Table 5-1 gives the proportions of children of hearing and deaf parents who use their hearing aids "always" or "almost always" at home and at school. In every comparison, hearing parents reported that their children use their hearing aids significantly more, regardless of whether they are deaf or hard of hearing and are at home or in school. However, this does not mean that deaf and hard of hearing parents ignore the benefits of hearing aids and speech training:

> *Both of my [deaf] kids had speech therapy at 6 months with [hearing] aids. I participated in a California program for free under [the John Tracy Clinic]. . . . My kids are better exposed to closed captions than my times. My mother put my hand on her [throat] to feel vibration. She interpreted everything. Today is better.* (Survey 313)

Table 5-1. Children Who Use Hearing Aids "Always" or "Almost Always"*

	At Home		At School	
	Hearing Parents	DF/HH Parents**	Hearing Parents	DF/HH Parents**
DF children	45.7%	16.0%	78.3%	52.0%
(n)	(105)	(25)	(106)	(25)
HH children	87.6%	56.3%	96.6%	56.3%
(n)	(154)	(16)	(146)	(16)

*Excluded are nonresponses, children with cochlear implants, and those using auditory trainers at school.

**One or both parents deaf or hard of hearing.

The big step is to make certain that she learns the speech and language at a certain time. Since the language development is important at early age. So that means extra responsibility for me to make sure she does not lag in language development in later life. . . . At [a] certain degree of deafness, I don't think [hearing loss] would be a problem for family communication, but [parents] should give a child a chance to hear or whatever enables the child to understand through communication because the world is full of hearing people. They need to build a bridge to the hearing world. (Survey 71)

Despite this parent's commitment to the importance of speech and language, her hard of hearing daughter was fitted with hearing aids only at 6 years of age. Asked about this delay, the mother responded:

Because of several reasons. First of all, at early age, hearing screening was . . . not most accurate. Secondly is that she was able to hear without the hearing aids at that time, only that we have to speak a little louder like a special amp [in] the phone that increase[s] the sound. And thirdly, she was young and aggressive that she played around at preschool as the hearing aids are so expensive and didn't want to take the risk for any loss, etc. . . . When she entered her first grade we realized that [she] was having some difficulty of understanding speech and noise background with lots of kids, so that's where we bought it and started at the age of 6. (Survey 71)

Another mother encouraged her son to use his hearing aids even though he resisted. When he moved to a school that placed less emphasis on auditory skills, she was less active in promoting hearing aid use:

He doesn't have the speech skills because when he was [at the local public school] he would be in audiology and speech and all that, but it didn't help at all and, um, myself as a mother . . . I felt it was really important for him to wear his hearing aids every day, but he just didn't want to. So I kept encouraging him to do that, but now he just doesn't wear them at all. He's used to not wearing them now. Now that he's at [the residential school], he doesn't take on the responsibility to remember to wear his hearing aids every day. So he really doesn't wear them at all now. (Survey 163)

This hard of hearing mother is particularly interested in her daughter's development of speechreading skills since the girl has a profound hearing loss (115 dB with hearing aids):

The school tested her periodically. I had asked that they test her with hearing aids on because I didn't want to be spending money on earmolds if she wasn't getting any benefit from them. She was just basically wearing them because her friends did. You know, and the hearing aids, the whistling was driving me crazy. . . . The feedback from the hearing aids because the earmolds didn't fit right.

[Asked what services she had found to be most helpful, the mother replied]: Well, at first, it was presenting different ideas on how to encourage speech development, well, not speech development so much because I really didn't think she would develop much speech because she is so deaf. Um, but I wanted her to lipread well. And to move her mouth according to the proper words that she was signing. So that's really what my focus is now. (Survey 260)

Educational Concerns

A common thread running through these interviews is a concern for education. As the excerpts relevant to hearing aids and speech training illustrate, some deaf parents are less concerned about those aspects of their children's experiences than are hearing parents. Concern about general academic education is a different matter. Asked about her concerns for her child after the identification of a hearing loss, this parent responded that education is of primary importance:

> *In the very beginning [we had no concerns], but as he entered school age our biggest concern was education. . . . I don't mean we were worried about how we were going to educate him. It was the issue of where we were going to send him for education, for, you and I know, schools for the deaf and mainstreamed programs are a big issue right now, and I was concerned there would be a small group of children his age in his class that he would still be challenged. We made sure he is being taught at grade level and is constantly challenged.* (Survey 27)

A hard of hearing mother emphasized the importance of English literacy:

> *I just think it's really important for a deaf child to read and to be good at reading and like to read. . . . So I guess I just get kind of crazy sometimes. . . . [This mother had worked as an interpreter in a school system that adopted SEE II in classrooms for deaf students.] I really objected to it [SEE II] and I couldn't live with it. So I quit my job. . . . I felt that it went against my beliefs and I just couldn't do that. I took the workshops and stuff and tried to learn the system, but I couldn't sleep at night because I disagreed with it so much. So I've been pursuing the bi-bi [bilingual-bicultural] approach. And I'm still not totally convinced it's the only way to go. I'm concerned about my children being fluent in written English, but I didn't think SEE II was what was going to make them fluent in written English . . .*
>
> *I have two brothers and a sister who are deaf. One brother and sister are profoundly deaf, and they grew up in residential schools. And I have a brother that's hard of hearing who grew up in mainstream programs. And he of course is very fluent in English and likes to read, whereas my other*

two siblings that are profoundly deaf, they're proficient enough in English, but neither one really reads for pleasure. And I don't want that for my children. I want them to read for pleasure. I want them to understand what they read and to learn from what they read. . . . I guess what I'm trying to promote for them is the desire to be proficient in written English. (Survey 260)

The next mother had specific expectations for her deaf child and appreciated information about general child development from an early intervention program:

I think their focus was more on the hearing child . . . and what was normal for them. I wanted that because I didn't want what was normal for the deaf. I wanted what was normal for [hearing] people. (Survey 261)

Actively engaged in a parent group at her daughter's school, this mother is concerned about teachers' expectations for deaf children:

We have a parent group at [a state residential school] that's, um, you know, actively trying to encourage the school to be more on the level of the hearing schools and promoting a curriculum that is the same to teach our deaf children as if they're normal and not "Oh, they're deaf, they can't do this or we don't expect that." I mean their expectations can be too low. Some of our teachers have been there for so long that I don't think they know what normal is any more. . . . We're just trying to be supportive in that area and encourage them to keep up their expectations of our children. We're concerned about their reading level. So many of us know deaf adults who are in very menial-type jobs, and we don't want that for our kids. We want them to have an opportunity to excel and have decent jobs. And starting with the deaf school itself, so many of the administration are hearing and very few deaf in high-level jobs there. I'm really disappointed about that. I would like to see them hire more qualified deaf adults, and they are telling me that there aren't more. Well, why is that? Because the education isn't so great that they're not putting out qualified deaf adults. And so that's kind of what we're working on. (Survey 260)

Another parent echoes these concerns about teachers' low expectations:

They need to change the way the teachers think. The way they teach needs to be equivalent to the way the hearing kids, what the hearing kids have to learn. It needs to be exactly the same. . . . . The deaf kids need to be educated equally to the hearing. Not lower their expectations for the deaf kids but keep it on an even keel with the hearing. (Survey 163)

Concerns for the future are linked to concerns about current educational practices:

My kids will have good education because I want them to succeed in the real world without help. (Survey 313)

Social Concerns

Educational concerns and social concerns are inextricably combined for many deaf parents. The proportions of students attending special schools have declined: In the 1973–1974 school year, 54% attended residential or day schools for deaf children, compared to 30% in 1997–1998 (Moores, 2001). Like the parents quoted here, many deaf parents choose to send their children to state residential schools rather than to mainstream programs. Gallaudet's annual survey showed that, from 1986 to 1996, residential school placement declined overall from 37% to 31%. However, among students with deaf parents, almost twice that percentage were in a residential placement, and the decline in the 10-year period was minimal: 62% in 1986 compared to 60% in 1996 (Holden-Pitt, 1997). Deaf people who are members of the Deaf community view the state residential schools as a primary transmitter of Deaf culture and regret the decline of their influence (Padden, 1996; Padden & Humphries, 1988). This and other changes mean that "the classic school for deaf children of a generation ago no longer exists" (Padden, 1996, p. 90).

Parents of deaf children often feel that educational placement decisions present a conflict between academic and social needs. Public school programs sometimes place a solitary deaf student among many hearing classmates, a situation that may lead to social isolation. Several mothers voiced these concerns:

> [H]e went into the infant program when he was 18 months, and he stayed at that school until he was 5 years old. Then he was mainstreamed, and he was the only deaf child in the classroom, and his language level was so high that he didn't really fit into the deaf program. So he was mainstreamed for 1 year in kindergarten, and he started to complain because, um, he didn't have any peers. There was no socialization because all of the kids in mainstream class were hearing. So he just wasn't happy. So I tried to help him, but within this community there just weren't peers of his age at his level. . . . So I made the decision that it would be best for him to transfer him to [the state residential school]. And he started first grade there, and he's been there all along. And right now he's in third grade there, and he has many peers there, and he's much happier. (Survey 163)

> It is good for her to attend deaf school instead of mainstream school because of activities, social life, the group understand that deaf school is best for her than mainstream school. (Survey 177)

> [Mainstreaming is] very difficult for the child itself—very isolated, not able to be around with hearing people. The child has an interpreter which are not always good signer. Not able to play in sports. (Survey 316)

Parents also expressed concerns about declining enrollments and successive closings or threats of phasing out state residential schools:

[Deaf parents] are worried about the children in the future, about the education since the deaf schools are shutting down or cut down the money from government. . . . We are worried about it. We need to watch the school and the government. We need to fight if [we see that happening]. (Survey 177)

The transmission of Deaf culture is an important value for many deaf parents:

The Deaf Community for Deaf Children, that organization, called DCDC, they were established a few years ago . . . and it's a volunteer group that goes to [her son's school], and the reason they go is . . . these are deaf adults that go to serve as a role model, so the kids can look up to them. And the kids see the adults signing in ASL and feel a connection with them. And they socialize with the kids, and there's a lot of communication going on. It's a wonderful benefit for the children. And these adults show the children that they can get a job, they can become a teacher, they can work at the post office, they can be a secretary. They can be a doctor or a lawyer, you know, whatever. (Survey 163)

Childhood experiences in a hearing family shape feelings about educational settings, as this mother relates:

My parents didn't sign at all. They believed strongly in oralism, the oral program, and we lived in a small town. . . . So they put me in an oral program, and it just didn't work because I had no language. I didn't have my parent's model as a first language . . . They would show me pictures, that was it. That was the only thing I knew. I didn't talk at all, and then when I was 9 years old, I learned how to read . . . but from infant to 9 years of age, I never sat down with my parents or . . . well, for example, at dinner time, we'd all sit down, and we would never sit together and communicate. Well . . . the rest of the family communicated except me. I wouldn't join in at dinner. I had no idea what stories they were telling, things that were going on. I had no idea. Until I was 9. Then my parents thought they should put me in a school for the deaf. . . . And that was [when] I was 9. And it was just an eye-opener. There was all these children there signing . . . but I had no language and I was completely lost. . . . So I started learning sign. I started off just learning a few signs. Until I was 15 years old. So from 9 to 15, it really took a long time to learn and pick up all of the signs. I learned all of the language from my friends. . . . On weekends when I would go home there was no communication at all. When I went back to [school] I was thrilled to go back because then I could start communicating and enjoying myself again. . . . [M]y mother —the two of us can still only write notes. That's all. So you know my arm is just tired by the time we finish talking to each other.

[Interviewer: That must be very painful and frustrating.] Oh yes, it was. It left a huge, huge mark on me. Huge, yes, it hurt me a lot. Yes. And that's the reason why I want to do so much for my son and be involved so much with him. And I feel like I owe that to him. (Survey 163)

Satisfaction with Early Services

Deaf parents were generally less satisfied than hearing parents with early services for their children, as their survey responses reflect. Interview responses help to explain those results:

I think that they understood my needs pretty well. It was OK, but I wouldn't say it was wonderful by any means. No. (Survey 163)

I would have liked to have had some guidance in terms of discipline. Um, I would have liked to have had parenting classes to learn how to discipline, so I could be involved in that. . . . It wasn't anything serious at all, but just I would have liked to have had something like that. . . . My husband is deaf also and works full time, and he supports the family. So my husband isn't really sure how to respond to different problems that are going on. . . . So really I don't get much support from him. So I just kind of have to roll up my sleeves and say "This is what you need to do." Like if he [our son] needs speech therapy. It would have been nice to have a mentor to help me . . . if I wanted to discuss things with them or what was going on at school . . . someone that I could have talked to about these things. Because I've never had a mentor . . . and also the same for my hearing daughter, too. I would have liked to have had a mentor to sit down and discuss things that were going on with her as well. (Survey 163)

However, other parents had positive reactions to their services. One parent said simply, "The program is awesome" (Survey 177). Others gave additional details:

The IEP [Individualized Educational Plan] was helpful [and] auditory and speech training, for we were unable to provide him with help in that area. . . . They had much to do with language development. They helped him with auditory discrimination, speech development, and building his self-confidence. Now this may be a little off the point, but I want to mention [that I] know the school is not solely responsible for the child's education or personal growth. The parents and family of the child [are] really responsible, but I want to add that [the school] has been very helpful in supporting this area. (Survey 27)

Deaf parents themselves are sometimes asked to serve as mentors for hearing parents with deaf children. Some intervention programs are built around the use of deaf parents as mentors (Mohay, 2000; Watkins, Pittman, & Walden, 1998). One interviewed deaf parent felt this experience was rewarding. Asked whether the program personnel had been sensitive to her needs, this parent replied:

Yes, yes, they also told me I helped them a lot, too, as far as just some of the things I was doing with [daughter]. They videotaped and, I guess, got some ideas or something. That's what I was told from a workshop they gave. But it was just helpful for me to have that time to spend alone with her and not be involved in everything else that is going on. You know, work and housework, bills, and that kind of thing. (Survey 260)

Although the next mother is generally positive, she has a suggestion for improving services to deaf parents:

I think a lot of the problem is that the hearing professionals that I know that work with the deaf infants is that they're not really proficient in sign. So, many of us, I mean our play group, our parent group, have interpreters because these people can't really sign fluently. Um, and I haven't really seen the deaf parents complain about that. They're so—usually—very tolerant because they do get such good services for their children, which is what they are there for. And I've never seen them complain, but I think there would be a better relationship between them if [the professionals] were more proficient in sign. (Survey 260)

Conclusion

As the social, economic, and legal status of deaf people in the United States has improved, deaf people have become increasingly confident about their parenting abilities, and their efforts as energetic and informed advocates for their children's education have accelerated. Deaf parents' concerns for their deaf children are similar to those of hearing parents. However, for most, hearing loss is not only expected but may even be welcomed as a familiar condition with which they are well prepared to cope. They urge professionals to become more proficient in sign language and to provide early contact with Deaf culture for both parents and children.

Chapter 6

Cochlear Implant Stories: Huge Decisions

Really, it's up to the parent. I mean, they [professionals] *could say "OK, we advise you to go ahead with this implant." But it was a huge thing and there was no guarantee. We were the ones who had to make the decision, nobody else could.* (Survey 80)

Parents' decisions to have cochlear implant surgery for their deaf child may be among the most difficult and important they will ever make. A medical doctor involved with implant surgery wrote the following: "This decision is often difficult . . . since it involves major surgery, some degree of pain and risk, significant financial obligations, years of rehabilitation, and as yet somewhat unpredictable results" (Cohen, 1997, p. 38). Despite these difficulties, 44 parents (11%) responding to the NPP survey opted for the procedure. An additional 24 children (6%) had been evaluated for the surgery, and 32 others (8%) had been considered for it. Thus, one quarter of the 404 parents responding to the survey had either considered the surgery or gone ahead with it. A survey of more than 4,000 children attending public education programs in Texas (1991–1992) showed that 13% of 6-year-olds and 7% of 7-year-olds had implants (Allen, Rawlings, & Remington, 1993). Data for all of the age groups in Gallaudet's annual survey show 3% of children with implants for 1994–1995. Between 1993 and 1995 the number of children with implants increased by 63% (Schildroth & Hotto, 1996).

Background on Cochlear Implants for Children

Several implant systems have been tested with clinical populations since the first single-channel 3M/House device received Food and Drug Administration (FDA) approval in 1983 (Nevins & Chute, 1996). Currently, the most widely used implant is the Nucleus 22-channel, developed in Australia and approved by the FDA in 1990 as safe and effective for children age 2 years and older. The manufacturers report that 40,000 people worldwide have received this device (Cochlear Corporation, 2002). Research performed under a 5-year contract with the U.S. National Institutes of Health "showed no cause for concern" for implant surgery with children younger than 2 years of age (Clark, 1999, p. 4), and a number of younger children have been implanted with no ill effects reported (Rizer & Burkey, 1999; Szagun, 2000). The Nucleus 24 Contour has been approved by the FDA for children age 12 months and older (Spencer, Christiansen, & Leigh, 2002). Implants have been approved for 8-month-olds in Germany but not in the United States (Calderon & Greenberg, 2000). Although not approved for use by children, a cochlear implant was recently developed for adults with partial deafness and high-frequency losses (Meadow-Orlans, 2001).

A cochlear implant system is composed of both internal and external components. An external microphone picks up the auditory signal and transmits it to connecting cables. These go to a speech processor that is placed either behind the ear or in a case worn on the body and that analyzes, filters, and codes signals that it then sends to a transmitting antenna. The antenna is held in place by a magnet located under the skin behind the ear. This internal magnet receives the sound signals and transmits them to the implanted electrode array that transmits information to the auditory nerve (Allum, 1996; Clark, Cowan, & Dowell, 1997).

Characteristics of NPP Implanted Children and Their Parents

The 44 children with cochlear implants whose parents responded to the survey received their devices from 1991 to 1996 and were between 2 and 6 years of age. This chapter includes quotations from interviews with 10 parents: 9 by telephone and 1 in a focus group. Compared to survey children without implants, those with implants were more likely to be girls, to

Table 6-1. Characteristics of Children with Implants (n = 44) and without Implants (n = 360)

	With Implants		Without Implants	
	%	(n)	%	(n)
Sex				
Girls	56	(23)	42	(151)
Boys	44	(18)	58	(205)
Hearing Level[a]				
Deaf	79	(33)	43	(147)
Hard of hearing	21	(9)	57	(196)
Additional Conditions				
None	72	(31)	68	(237)
One or more	28	(12)	33	(114)
Number of Siblings				
None or one	73	(32)	58	(207)
Two or more	27	(12)	42	(149)
Racial/Ethnic Group				
White, non-Hispanic	75	(33)	66	(235)
Other	25	(11)	34	(120)
Mother's Education[b]				
Some college	74	(32)	55	(195)
No college	26	(11)	45	(157)

[a]Chi square = 19.2; df = 65.9; p = .001

[b]Chi square = 5.67; df = 1; p = .02

See Appendix C for a glossary of statistical terms and abbreviations used in tables.

be deaf rather than hard of hearing, to have no additional conditions, and to have fewer siblings. Their mothers were less likely to be from minority groups and more likely to have some college education (Table 6-1).

Some of these differences are undoubtedly linked to characteristics (e.g., hearing level, presence of additional conditions) of children deemed good or poor candidates for benefit from an implant. Others may well be linked to economic advantage or disadvantage and the high cost of implant surgery and postsurgery rehabilitation. These NPP data, as well as those from other sources, show that privileged children are more likely than poor children to receive implants (Allen, Rawlings, & Remington, 1993; Schildroth

& Hotto, 1996). We agree that "the underrepresentation of racial and ethnic groups is a serious ethical concern" (Christiansen & Leigh, 2002, p. 307).

Parents Discuss Cochlear Implants

Interviewed parents of implanted children discussed the issues of eligibility for surgery, the high cost of implants, surgical hazards, opposition from
the Deaf community, and the parents' motivations for seeking the implantation for their children. These interviews also covered children's initial
reactions to the implant, postsurgical training, evaluation of benefits, and
support that parents received relevant to implantation.

Considerations Prior to Surgery

Eligibility for Surgery

Several reports provide guidelines for identifying children who are good
candidates for a successful implant, but surgeons are not required to follow these recommendations (Calderon & Greenberg, 1997). At the time
the NPP survey children received their implants, it was generally believed
that a child should be at least 2 years old and profoundly deaf (unable to
receive significant assistance from a hearing aid), have no major disability,
and be a good candidate for the significant habilitation required for the
implant to make a difference in their sound and speech perception. No
NPP child received an implant before the age of 2 years (average age was
43.5 months). Half were implanted before the age of 38 months.

The following family's experience with two different centers may
reflect differences in adherence to guidelines:

*When Mary was maybe 1 or 2 [years old], we made an appointment
with . . . an excellent ear doctor [who] does cochlear implants. . . . He
advised against doing the surgery because Mary wasn't deaf enough. . . .
He said come back every year. So we went back a couple more times, just
to check. And then I went to a meeting . . . [where a woman] from the
[Y] Clinic was . . . talking about cochlear implants. . . . I talked to her
afterward, and she said, "Well, why don't you bring Mary up for an evaluation?" . . . They did the evaluation and said, "Well, as far as I can tell,*

she meets the guidelines." I guess the guidelines were loosened at some
point. (Survey 30)

Although eligibility guidelines discouraged implanting children with additional conditions, 28% of NPP children with implants had some condition in addition to hearing loss. This is the same proportion as that reported for a large (n = 1,020) survey of U.S. and Canadian implanted children (Hasenstab, 1997). Among the NPP implant children, 9 had one additional condition, 2 had two, and 1 had three conditions. Four were identified as developmentally delayed; 3 with attention deficit disorder; 2 with behavior problems; 1 each with impaired vision, epilepsy, and a learning disability; and 4 with unidentified conditions.

One mother described the experience of a child with multiple disabilities known to her who had received an implant:

Not all children are candidates. And we have one in particular here who wasn't a candidate but got it anyway . . . and it's just been very . . . umm . . . frustrating for her. (Survey 101)

Another mother described her son's behavior, which had initially prevented his being considered for an implant. He had been in an auditory verbal program for 2 years, a strict oral training regimen:

We had some really bad times [about age 4] where he would spit at the student therapists or he would spend the whole time in the corner. We later found out that he had ADD [attention deficit disorder], too. . . . They said he should be a candidate for cochlear implants. [The auditory verbal specialist] had also told me this, but he had too many behavioral issues, and I know he would [have thrown] it over a chandelier and be swinging with it at that time when he was younger. (Survey 286)

The High Cost of Implant Surgery

Many families cannot afford the expensive surgery, although some receive public assistance, and others have medical insurance covering all or part of the cost. Of parents responding to another survey, 58% received full insurance coverage for the surgery and implant programming, while about 40% had coverage for habilitation therapy (Christiansen & Leigh, 2002). The cost is $40,000 to $50,000 for the initial surgery. Postimplant rehabilitation can involve a team of doctors, speech therapists, and others working with a child for several years at a cost of perhaps $20,000 per year (Marschark, Lang, & Albertini, 2002). This undoubtedly excludes many families. One interview study found that an important secondary consideration for the implant decision was the availability of insurance coverage (Kluwin & Stewart, 2000). High costs discourage consideration:

I saw a "60 Minutes" [television] special [featuring a child with an implant], and I was really interested. So I talked to his teacher . . . and she . . . told me . . . she would get some information on it. And she came back and told me that the insurance didn't pay for it. . . . And the operation was like $40,000, and I knew that was not possible. Not at that time anyway. (Survey 185)

Another mother is grateful for the financial assistance that enabled her child to have the surgery:

One of the big services we got that's available in [our state] is we got funding for all the stuff . . . right from the beginning. There's a program called the Crippled Children's, which is funded by the state for special needs kids. . . . They paid for the implant, which was $40,000, and they paid for all her hearing therapy. I mean, we've hardly spent anything. And all the services, of course, are provided by the schools. So that's been a huge thing that's really helped us, a big service. . . . Our theory has been all along, even though some of the stuff costs a lot of money and it's kind of a stretch, the more we invest in her now, the better it's going to be. She'll be a better citizen, she'll be less dependent, she'll be able to contribute more, she'll be more able to take care of herself. I mean, all these things we're doing for her now will make her a very independent, well-rounded person when she grows up. (Survey 80)

This mother's justification of the time, effort, and money expended on her daughter mirrors the conclusion of a cost-benefit study. A comparison of the educational placements and services provided to deaf students with and without cochlear implants showed that those with implants and a 1-year habilitation program were more likely to enter regular public school programs and to use less special education support. The authors estimate that, from kindergarten through grade 12, savings ranged from $30,000 to $200,000 per pupil (Francis, Koch, Wyatt, & Niparko, 1999). Opponents of cochlear implants, on the other hand, argue that the large amounts of private and public monies spent in this way might be better spent providing conventional support to all deaf and hard of hearing children and families (Hindley, 2000).

Motivations for Surgery

Decisions may be related to values regarding the ability to communicate, academic achievement, social life, and emotional well-being (Steinberg et al., 2000). The usual parental goal is to enable a child to understand speech and to produce intelligible oral/spoken language. One survey showed that 52% of parents decided on an implant for "ease in development and use of oral spoken language." Another 25% checked "safety/environmental awareness" as the main reason (Christiansen & Leigh, 2002). An interview study reports that parents' most important reason was "a desire . . . to have a child who might function as a hearing person" (37%); for an additional 26%, a major factor was their own frustration with "the child's communication skills" (Kluwin & Stewart, 2000, p. 29).

Interviewed parents expressed a wide range of motivations, including a desire to give their deaf child "every opportunity" (Spencer, 2000a). "Because [implants are] new and very technical, expectations by those considering them may be unreasonably high" (Kampfe et al., 1993, p. 298). Before surgery is performed, doctors usually caution parents about the limitations of implants:

Of course, the doctor would only say, "She'll hear a bus coming, she'll hear horns and sirens and warnings and the phone ring and syllables, at least, over the telephone." I really thought it would be more than that but

*you don't know how much more. And I didn't count on it being perfect
hearing. . . . We weren't naïve. . . . I just felt like she wanted to talk. . . .
She was born to talk. And she wasn't progressing greatly with what we
were doing. I believed it would really help her.* (Survey 30)

In the next example, a sudden and unexplained shift from partial to
profound deafness resulted in an immediate deterioration of a child's communication ability:

*Over one weekend, when she was almost 4, she lost all the rest of her
hearing. Just spontaneously, nobody knows why. She wasn't sick, nothing
happened, and it just all went. And needless to say that was very traumatic, and everybody just flipped out, and she became very difficult to
communicate with, very difficult to manage behaviorally. She was a
mess. I was a mess. But because we were already being seen at the university, which had a big implant program, they fast-tracked us into that
program and jumped us ahead of kids who had been on the waiting list
because she was such a perfect candidate. She's very, very smart, very
determined to communicate. . . . So they were just thrilled to death to
think they'd have this sort of child who possibly could benefit greatly from
this thing. So they implanted her a few days after her fourth birthday.*
(Survey 80)

Another family felt they had "tried everything" before opting for
implant surgery:

*[When] Amy was about 10 months old, other children her age were
responding to their name and she didn't. So we started . . . testing her,
making loud noises behind her, and she just didn't respond. And so at 11
months the audiologist diagnosed it. And then we thought, "Well, put
tubes in her ears; that will fix it," and that didn't work. So I was fortunate*

to work in a company where Dr. [X] from [AAA Institute] was on the board of directors. He and another one of our board members were kind of instrumental in developing the cochlear implant. So that night I was in tears at work, and our [company] president said, "Well, we're calling Dr. [X] right now." I talked to him, and he said, "A cochlear implant is the way you need to go, but you know you've still got over a year before you can do that [to reach the age of eligibility]." So we said, "OK, we'll try hearing aids," but we know they're not gonna work. And so at 25 months she had the implant. (Survey 101)

For the following parent, academic achievement was a major motivating value:

When the teachers told us he was doing fine but he couldn't hear a thing, I said to my husband . . . this is the time we have to make a decision. Umm, he can get through kindergarten and the first grade, but when it comes to philosophy and economics . . . he is not going to be able to. It's not going to be easy for him; it's just going to get more and more frustrating. We are asking him to run a race on one leg. Either we give him the benefit of the full power of hearing as much as he can or we switch to a TC school. (Survey 286)

For another parent, concerns about social issues in the future were important:

Our biggest concern was she'll never have a prom date! [laughter] Which is funny because I was talking to another mother of a little girl who is deaf and that was her [concern], too. My biggest concern was that people weren't going to like her and weren't going to accept her. . . . And she's got boyfriends already, so [laughter] I don't think I have to worry about a prom date. (Survey 101)

Opposition from the Deaf Community

The decision to implant was sometimes made in a conflict-laden atmosphere that is similar to the climate within deaf education, adding further stress to a parent's already heavy load (Meadow-Orlans, 2002b). Some members of the Deaf community and some hearing advocates have been outspoken in their opposition to cochlear implants, seeing them as a threat to the community's existence (Lane, 1992; Mowl, 1996). Responses from a few representatives of the medical community have been equally harsh. One physician referred to hearing advocates as "rescuers," some of whom have "misled the Deaf community, ignored the cost of deafness and castigated the . . . values of the American family" (Balkany, 1995, p. 5).

However, Moores, a long-time researcher in deaf education, believes that "we are starting to address some of the most critical questions concerning implants in a balanced way" (2000, p. 3). This assessment is supported by a revised position statement on cochlear implants that the National Association of the Deaf (NAD) released in January 2001. In contrast to an earlier position paper, this specifically welcomes implant users to the Deaf community and recognizes the right of parents to make the implant decision for a child. A consistent theme throughout the lengthy statement is that cochlear implantation is a technology that represents a tool to be used with some forms of communication and that is not a cure for deafness (NAD Cochlear Implant Committee, 2001, p. 14).

One hopes that the changing atmosphere will decrease the future likelihood of experiences such as the following one that a member of a parent focus group reported:

It wasn't an easy decision. We had no idea if we were making the right decision. . . . We went through a lot of controversy with the Deaf community. You know, somehow people heard that I was going to do this. It's like a grapevine or something. Harassing phone calls and . . . [some] professionals . . . [said] "Are you sure you want to do this?" (Focus Group 3)

Another parent attended a camp designed for children with implants and their families where some of the other parents reported similar experiences with members of the Deaf community:

A lot of the parents that were in the group said that they had flak from the Deaf communities. That "the child is deaf, leave 'em deaf." "Deaf is beautiful" or whatever. (Survey 76)

Decision Not to Implant

Although members of the Deaf community did not influence them, two mothers participating in focus groups had considered implants for their children but had dismissed the possibility for different reasons:

We visited a family whose child had a cochlear implant because my husband was really interested. I was not. I said, "There's nothing wrong with his brain. I don't want to make him hearing if he's not." To me it's just not a natural thing to do. They showed us videotapes of what he had to go through— hours and hours of instruction. So I pretty much convinced my husband. If [my son] wants to try it when he grows up, that's fine. (Focus Group 1)

We looked into a cochlear implant, and I just thought it was ridiculous to have all these wires hanging from a 3-year-old's head. You'd have to replace those things, and the doctor explained that the sounds he would be hearing would not be the sounds that we hear. (Focus Group 1)

The Risk of Surgery

Surgery for a cochlear implant entails some pain and risk. Although these may be minimal, parents will probably factor them into their decision. Two families were concerned about the risks of surgery; a third continues to worry about long-term effects:

Well, surgery is surgery, and I didn't want to put her through anything that I felt was extremely risky, which we were assured it was not even considered even major surgery. . . . The whole time . . . she was in there, we were sweating. Not because of . . . any anesthesia problem. You know, kids go in for tonsils and end up dying. . . . We didn't want to think of things like that, but it's always on your mind. (Survey 226)

I am a nurse and . . . I know . . . the risks of surgery, and, yeah, up to the last minute we were wondering should we do it, and my husband was ready to pull him out at the last minute . . . mostly because of the anesthesia and him being such a little guy. (Survey 286)

I have to admit—and I've never read that this would happen—but I don't like the idea of electrical impulses in her head. I worry that some day when she's 50, she'll have brain cancer. I've never heard of that happening. I just have to hope. That's a risk, and I don't know how realistic a risk. (Survey 30)

Postsurgery Experiences

Initial Reaction to the Implant

Parents expressed some concerns about their child's initial reaction to the new experience of sound and considerable trepidation about their response. Two who described this introduction to sound through the implant reported that their children had very different experiences: One had an intense dislike of the appliance; the other expressed pleasure:

She hated it at first. After the surgery [at 26 months], we brought her home, and she had this big bandage on her head, and she was in her crib, and I heard this horrible ruckus. And we went in there, and the bandage was beside the door, and her crib was totally across the room. She had taken that thing off and chucked it to get rid of it. But when we had it turned on (it took us 45 minutes before she would let us put the processor on), she just hated it. She had been in a nice little quiet world and all of a sudden—chaos! But she got used to it. Now she'll take a bath and want to put it back on so she can listen to the TV or talk on the phone. So she doesn't like to not hear any more. Unless we're fussing at her and she will take the magnet off and close her eyes. She's learned that! (Survey 101)

[The postsurgical training] was very brief. The audiologist explained how to operate it, what signs to look for that he may not have accepted it, because [for] some kids, it's the first time they're hearing sound, and it is probably a scary thing for them. But at that time Sam was almost 5 years old, so he was a little older than the other little kids, and he took it fine. [When they attached the processor], he just smiled. When we called his name, he turned and looked. It's just a great experience! (Survey 185)

Other researchers who interviewed parents of 63 implanted children, ages 4 to 18, report the following:

> Their child did in fact respond in some way to sound in the first mapping session; only three families said that there was no response at all. The most common initial reaction was crying, and about half of the parents said that their child appeared to be scared or frightened when sounds were first heard. . . . A couple of parents said that their child was overwhelmed at the initial activation, whereas another parent said that their child signed "weird" when asked to describe what the sound was like. (Christiansen & Leigh, 2002, p. 140)

Postsurgical Training to Utilize the Implant

All of the accounts of cochlear implantation, for children or adults, emphasize the importance of postsurgical habilitation to ensure a beneficial outcome (Calderon & Greenberg, 1997). Some parents may decide to go ahead with the implant surgery without understanding the postimplant time commitment, which can contribute to a lack of success (Kluwin & Stewart, 2000). For example, the program at the University of Iowa Hospitals and Clinics involves frequent visits for child and parents, informal speech perception training, parental diaries of the child's listening and speaking behaviors, and parental training in facilitating the child's speech perception. "[The children] learn how to initiate a conversation, how to practice good speaking behaviors, how to organize a message before speaking . . . how to detect a failure in communication, and how to repair conversational breakdowns" (Tye-Murray & Kelsay, 1993, p. 26). Most of the parents in this study had a thorough grounding in post-surgery requirements:

[The doctor in a southeastern city] had told us that his office did not pro-vide rehabilitation. He could do the surgery, but we would be on our own for rehabilitation. . . . I had read a book that basically said if a doctor would . . . not provide rehabilitation, that was frowned upon. The sug-gestion was that it was unethical to do the surgery without also providing the necessary follow-up care—and we were concerned about that. And when we went to [a second city], of course we asked about rehabilitation. They have a staff of audiologists and speech pathologists and all of the rehabilitation-type services that a cochlear implant patient would need. So we chose to stay with the [second city] doctor. . . . Rehabilitation is just too important to overlook. (Survey 224)

Another mother describes a difficult postsurgical path:

[After the surgery, when we started rehabilitation] . . . well, she ended up getting five Barbie dolls as bribes by the time we got her going with it because I did not know what to do. I thought, "Oh no, we've gone through all this, and she's never going to wear it." So I called someone at [a uni-versity clinic] because I think they do a lot of implants with children. And the woman there said (that's all I remember her saying), "Bribery works." And it did. (Survey 30)

To Sign or Not to Sign

The old oral-manual controversy was apparently laid to uneasy rest in the mid-1970s, when Total Communication became the communication mode of choice for most parents and educational programs. The growing acceptance of cochlear implants has revived that controversy, with some implant centers strongly opposing parents' use of sign language with their implanted children. Like the old controversy, this is based on the "least effort" argument: A child will prefer the mode that he or she finds easier (and it is assumed that signing is easier than speech and speechreading for those with a severe or profound hearing loss). A more moderate approach, in programs where parents are not asked to abandon signing, may "encourage parents to rely more on the auditory signal for communication" (Tye-Murray & Kelsay, 1993, p. 24). It is possible that as implant teams have acquired more experience, their proscriptions against signing have lessened. The Listening Center at Johns Hopkins University advises parents that a visual system in use before implantation "should not be terminated immediately following activation of the cochlear implant" (Christiansen & Leigh, 2002, p. 155).

Parents' decisions about the use of sign language vary widely, as do the conclusions of published research. Studies of speech perception show both better and worse performance by child implant users exposed to manual communication (Meyer, Svirsky, Kirk, & Miyamoto, 1998; Miyamoto, Osberger, Robbins, Myres, & Kessler, 1993).

About three quarters of the NPP mothers and 65% of the fathers of implanted children report that they use some signs or cues with their children, not significantly different from those whose children do not have implants. Interviewed mothers provide important insights about the use of sign language:

> It's really speech alone. . . . [We sign] some words . . . that we all learned when she was real little, like "who" and "where" and "bathroom." One-word signs that we can do. But we're really not signing to her at home. She is signing at school because she's sharing an interpreter. She has an interpreter with another little deaf child who is all sign. So Amy has really picked up on sign. She's coming home daily and telling us we're wrong, signing it wrong. And she's doing both. But outside of school, she's just oral. (Survey 101)

> Well, since she's had the cochlear implant, we try to talk to her first. And if she doesn't get it, I'll say it slower, and if she [still] doesn't get it, we'll sign. It's not that strict, but generally speaking, I try to encourage her to hear it. But she still doesn't hear it a lot of the time, so we would have been lost without sign language. She would've been lost, I dhink. And she still relies on it to some extent. We've talked to some people who advised

us not to teach her sign language. And that if she did sign, she wouldn't speak. But as we tried to do that, she just wasn't there. She wasn't getting any of it. I think we felt like her language was more important than that she be strictly a speaking person. And the ideas that she could start to develop at a young age were more important than that she just strictly speak. (Survey 30)

We thought we might learn sign language when she first lost all her hearing, but we didn't. The people we worked with [after] her cochlear implant had told us that it's better not to use sign language if she's going to rely on the cochlear implant. So at some point we may certainly let her exercise the choice to learn sign language, but right now that would not be compatible with her cochlear implant as we understand it. And she communicates very well. The speech therapist is ready to let her out of speech therapy. She's mastered the "s" and the "z" and the "sh" and the sounds that are very hard to hear with hearing aids. So she's oral. And she reads lips like a champ. (Survey 224)

Evaluation of Benefits

Most published studies of children's postimplant performance describe speech perception and production in response to closed-set testing (picture identification or sentence completion), which provides context (Marschark, 2000; Szagun, 2000). Although parents expect their deaf child to function like one who is hard of hearing, most studies report only modest gains.

One representative study of speech perception showed that children with implants achieved higher scores than children without implants and with 101–110 dB hearing loss and approached scores for children with 90–100 dB hearing loss, where both groups of nonimplant children used hearing aids (Meyer, Svirsky, Kirk, & Miyamoto, 1998; see also Geers & Moog, 1995). Only a few studies of language comprehension and production have been undertaken. One ($n = 25$) showed that "the cochlear implant facilitates children's ability to perceive and comprehend bound morphemes" (Spencer, Tye-Murray, & Tomblin, 1998).[1] Another (*n* = 10) analyzed spontaneous speech samples and found that most implanted children produce multiword utterances and acquire considerable verb inflectional morphology (Szagun, 2000; see also Tomblin, Spencer, Flock, Tyler, & Gantz, 1999).[2] As several researchers have observed, children vary greatly in their ability to utilize an implant effectively. Some of the factors contributing to this variability include age at implantation, elapsed time since surgery was performed, consistency of implant use, hearing level before surgery, and consistency of postsurgery training (Tomblin et al., 1999; Tye-Murray & Kelsay, 1993).

The author of one recent and extensive review of implant studies concludes that the positive outcomes greatly exceed the negative ones: The "average" outcome is one in which sounds are detected 90% of the time, but spoken language is correctly identified less than 50% of the time. Most implantees have only limited use of the telephone (Spencer, 2002). "Unfortunately for both users and investigators, outcome variability is so great that it is difficult to make any good generalizations at this point" (Marschark, Lang, & Albertini, 2002, p. 55).

A parent's evaluation of a child's cochlear implant depends to a great extent on his or her prior expectations and the child's subsequent performance. The NPP survey form asked, "Are the [implant] results satisfactory?" Of those who responded, 67% said that the implant was "very satisfactory." Twelve said the implant was "not satisfactory"; nevertheless, two of these children still used it. The Gallaudet Research Institute survey (*n* = 439) utilized a 4-point scale of satisfaction: Of parents responding, 67% indicated they were "very satisfied" with their child's cochlear implant progress, and 39% were "very satisfied" with their child's development of spoken language skills (Christiansen & Leigh, 2002).

The following excerpts illustrate the NPP parents' perceptions of a "very satisfactory" outcome:

---

1. A *bound morpheme* is a grammatical unit that cannot stand alone but is always attached to a whole word (e.g., "-ness" in "deafness" or "un-" in "undo").
2. The ability to use verb tenses correctly (e.g., "He *went* yesterday." "I *go* today.").

It actually helped her. Although if we sign to her, I think she would just as soon go with that. [She doesn't really like] the apparatus. But it really has helped her speech tremendously. Although I'm sure it would have gotten better anyway. She goes to a dance class, and the dance teacher is amazed. When she started she really couldn't talk at all. She was 4. And now she can understand a lot of what is said. (Survey 30)

She has been a tremendous success story. It's been absolutely the most miraculous thing you can imagine. She's mainstreamed in school. She was in the hearing-impaired program from age 3 through kindergarten. And this year she's mainstreamed with a lot of extra help, but she's learning to talk. She has what they would classify more as a mild language delay now, but her speech is beautiful. I think of her more as just a normal kid. You deal with her the same way you do with all the other kids. Like, are we going to go to [the Brownie meeting] and which gymnastics class should she take—that sort of thing. (Survey 80)

She's very outgoing, and she does really well communicating with others. Particularly this year it's gotten to where people can understand her, and she can talk on the phone and order at fast-food restaurants, and we're very pleased with her progress. . . . We still have a lot of challenges with Amy, like we'll be riding in the car and she'll be in the back seat and it's constantly, "What? What? Look at me, Mom." But most of the conversation [is OK, even] if I'm not sitting there staring at her. Whereas if she was totally deaf and didn't hear anything, you'd have to be looking at her constantly or turn around and sign to her. It would be so much more difficult. But we've been so pleased with her implant. (Survey 101)

The most helpful thing was the cochlear implant. We saw tremendous changes as far as him hearing things that he couldn't hear with his aids. His aids never really helped him because he always received feedback no matter what . . . but the implant is great! . . . A couple of months after he was implanted, I [wondered], "Did I do this for my own selfish reasons, or did I do this to help Sam?" He was responding to his name more, he

was responding to different sounds he hadn't heard before, but it contin-
ues to be a slow process. But every time he goes back and gets tested, we
see that he does score better on the test, he scores higher. The implants are
not for every child. But I wouldn't change what I've done for nothing.
(Survey 185)

She's a very active child. She does what most every other 7-going-on-8-
year-old would do as far as schoolwork. She's mainstreamed in school.
She is an avid reader. You can't take books away from her. She's reading
in the bathtub right this minute. She's in Brownie Scouts, she is active in
church, she sings in the choir and goes to Sunday school and does every-
thing most kids do and plays with kids in the neighborhood. . . . She's
been in Girl Scout camp. She's an incredibly active, inquisitive, and (the
mother in me says) brilliant 7-year-old. My husband's impartial and he
thinks so, too. . . . She's pulled out of the classroom to work with the itin-
erant teacher a couple of times a week. They also pull her out for speech
therapy, but she's about to graduate from that. . . . We use speech. When
she's not wearing her speech processor that goes to her cochlear implant,
she reads lips. I had taken Cued Speech lessons, and we used it a little bit
a couple of years ago to distinguish between "tah" and "dah" and the "t"
and the "d" sounds she was having trouble with. But since she got the
cochlear implant and the speech processor she's distinguished very well,
and we haven't had to use the Cued Speech. (Survey 224)

Support for Parents

Support for parents has long been a cornerstone of early intervention services for deaf and hard of hearing children and their families (Meadow-Orlans & Sass-Lehrer, 1995). An English surgeon emphasized that parents of children with implants have even more critical needs for support than other parents of deaf children. He notes that "the acquisition of intelligible speech is vexingly slow and periods of parental disillusionment are commonplace" (O'Donoghue, 1996, p. 346P). Thus, the support of families in the years following implantation is necessary if they are to give their children sufficient encouragement in the use of their implant systems. As these systems became more complex, requiring increased tuning or mapping, the amount of time and therefore support required continued to increase (Quittner, Steck, & Rouiller, 1991). Parents responding to another survey reported that many professionals were involved in facilitating the child's use of the implant. These included an audiologist (95%), a surgeon (86%), a speech pathologist (75%), a psychologist (35%), a teacher of deaf children (34%), an educational consultant (20%), a social worker (10%), and other professionals (3%) (Christiansen & Leigh, 2002).

The NPP parents of children receiving implants felt they had received more support compared to other survey parents. Total scores on the Support Scale were significantly higher than scores of other parents. This difference was accounted for by higher scores (that is, greater perceived support) from parents, spouses' parents, and other extended family members. Interviewed parents expressed a great deal of gratitude for the professional help and support they had received:

> They've been very responsive as far as the speech therapy and the provision of hearing services. . . . I can speak for my experiences and other parents' experiences, too. If we have a question, we pick up the phone and call. And they've been really responsive. . . . I know basically what the rights are. I checked that out early, too, like Public Law 94-142 and the things that come after that: ADA and IDEA. I know how to invoke whatever rights we might need to invoke, but we haven't had to do any of that . . . We're just lucky. (Survey 224)

Another mother appreciated the personal attention as well as the professional expertise that accompanied her daughter's services:

> Of course we had a speech and language therapist, and they monitored her physical therapy stuff, but mostly it was the program. It was a very small group of kids all her own age, and the teacher just became kind of like an aunt. She showed up at the hospital right after the surgery. And

she's the one who we talked to on the phone almost every day. "How's Mimi doing? What's going on?" So it wasn't just a school setting. These were very, very involved teachers who were working outside with the kids. They'd come to all the birthday parties and [family gatherings]. The services were very good. (Survey 80)

Conclusion

Cochlear implant technology is moving so rapidly that it is impossible to predict future developments. The age at which surgery is approved for infants has decreased again and again. Much has been learned about post-surgical habilitation, and more and more children are evaluated and approved as potential candidates for the procedure. However, long-term effects, in terms of years rather than months, are still unknown. Today's children and their parents are the pioneers. Children in the future will benefit from their experiences.

Chapter 7

Minority Families: Wave of the Future

With Kimberley Scott-Olson

And, uh, my biggest concern was if he wanted to be president, I wanted him to be able to. Simply because I wanted him to have the same opportunities as my hearing children. (Survey 202)

The results of Census 2000 confirm the increasing diversity in the U.S. population (U.S. Census Bureau, 2001). Although respondents were for the first time given the opportunity to identify themselves in more than one racial category, 98% of all of the respondents chose only one category. The largest group reported White only (75%); the Black- or African American-only population represented 12% of the total. Asian was the third most-reported race (4%), and less than 1% reported American Indian or Alaska Native. Hispanics, who could put themselves in any racial category in the census, represented about 13% of the population. Forty-eight percent of those who identified themselves as Hispanic also identified as White only, while about 42% chose "some other race." The Hispanic population is projected to triple, from 31.4 million in 1999 to 98.2 million in 2050, making that the nation's largest minority group. The African American population is expected to rise by 70% during this same 50-year period.

The significance of these demographic shifts is underscored by the knowledge that ethnic and racial minorities are overrepresented in the deaf and hard of hearing communities compared to the general population (Gallaudet Research Institute, 2001). The Annual Survey of Deaf Children and Youth for 1999–2000 reveals that approximately 45% of deaf children are from an ethnic/racial minority group. The largest proportion is Hispanic (21%), followed by Black/African American (16%). Asian Pacific deaf children make up 4% of the population, and less than 1% are

Native American. White only, not Hispanic, constitute 55% of deaf children and youth.

This chapter explores the concerns and issues of minority families with deaf and hard of hearing children. Research that addresses this particular perspective is limited (Christensen, 2000; Mertens, 1998). The diversity in the current U.S. population, the census population projections, as well as the overrepresentation of minority groups in the deaf and hard of hearing population, increase the importance of examining views of parents with deaf and hard of hearing children from these groups.

Characteristics of Minority Families

In the NPP survey, 33% of the respondents were minority parents. This percentage was somewhat less than the 42% of minority families who responded to the Annual Survey of Deaf and Hard of Hearing Children and Youth that the Gallaudet Research Institute conducted at about the same time as the NPP survey in 1997 (Holden-Pitt & Diaz, 1998).

Twenty-one parents provided the qualitative data for this chapter. We interviewed 11 by telephone and 1 mother/father pair in person. Eight participated in one of the focus groups. We conducted the telephone interviews with 4 parents of African American children and 7 parents of mixed-race children. ("Mixed race" refers to children whose parents checked more than one race on the survey, e.g., Black and White, or White and Hispanic.) Of the 17 parents in the focus groups, 8 were minorities: 2 Asian, 2 Hispanic, and 4 African American. One of the parents was hard of hearing; all of the others had normal hearing.

Of the 20 children represented, 16 were boys and 4 were girls. Six parents described their children as hard of hearing, while 14 described their children as deaf.

The following characteristics could be determined only for the 11 families who participated in both the national survey and the telephone interviews. Four reported that the diagnosis of their child's hearing loss was delayed, and 1 reported the presence of a behavior problem; 2 children had cochlear implants, 8 had one or more siblings, and 5 had a disability as well as a hearing loss.

Several parents described their children as having a hearing loss and many good qualities such as being smart, determined, funny, able to draw very well, skilled in sports, good in math, and sensitive to the needs of others. Some parents balanced their positive descriptions with other personality characteristics that are also typical of young children, such as being stubborn. Three descriptions follow:

He's hearing impaired. It's profound in his right ear and moderate to profound on his left. So he wears two hearing aids, and he does sign, and he reads lips, and he's learning how to read. And that's about it. He's a sweet little boy. (Survey 334)

I'm proud of my son because he achieved a lot of stuff. When he was about 3 years old, he started learning sign, and he picked it up so quickly. He has a mind to learn so quick, and I'm just proud of him because he is determined to learn in school, and he wants to go to school, and he wants to learn. Plus I think I'm proud of him because he is smart and he is determined and that's what makes me proud of him. Because I know he is gonna get somewhere and be somebody. I know he is. (Focus Group 2)

You see them out there playing. I go to a park and I say, "Oh, he's not going to be able to demonstrate that he wants to play with the ball. Those kids are not going to let him in." Though, when they might not let him in, he does some flips or something. Basically, the whole group is over there with him. He's never had a problem. He goes to the park to this day. He just mingles right in. He demands your presence. . . . I mean, he just has that kind of, you know, where I can do something that you can do but better. (Focus Group 3)

Limitations

The data from the minority subgroups were limited with regard to language and inclusiveness of diverse populations. The Spanish translation of the national survey instrument was flawed, and interviews and focus groups were conducted in English. Therefore, the Hispanic participants were either relatively fluent in English or acquired assistance in responding to the survey.

Second, there is great diversity in country of origin, language skill, and immigration status within each ethnic or racial group. For example, the Hispanic population in the United States includes people from many Latin American countries, each with its own unique cultural traditions (Gerner de Garcia, 2000; Ramsey, 2000). Asian Americans have traditionally been from China, Japan, Korea, or the Philippines (Cheng, 2000). More recently, immigrants from countries such as Vietnam, Laos, and Cambodia, as well as from India and Pakistan, have increased dramatically. Our respondents are limited with respect to the diversity and number of minority groups they represent: No Native Americans and only two Asian countries are represented. Because the national survey did not include country of origin, that information is not available.

Given the small and diverse qualitative sample, it is possible neither to tease out nuances of experiences based on these dimensions of diversity nor to claim that what we present here is representative of the members of these populations in a statistical way. Nevertheless, the comments of the parents in this study provide insight into the experiences of some of the members of ethnic and racial minority groups who have children who are deaf and hard of hearing.

Themes

We have reported the interview data according to themes that emerged from the qualitative analysis of the transcripts. These themes include warning signs; circumstances of identification of hearing loss and parental responses; concerns about rights, discrimination, aspirations, and finances; support from extended family and siblings, religion, and professionals; communication at home and at school; and access to and satisfaction with services.

In many ways these parents' experiences mirror those of other parents with young deaf or hard of hearing children. Sometimes themes emerge that seem more specific to the parents' status as members of a minority group living in the dominant White culture. Such themes provide food for thought regarding implications for other families who find themselves in similar circumstances, as well as for the professionals who serve them. The overlapping in themes found between the White and non-White parents underscores the universal nature of response to childhood deafness. Even though race and ethnicity are critically important dimensions, parents of deaf and hard of hearing children share many other characteristics and experiences. The commonality, as well as the uniqueness of minority group membership, provides a more complete picture of these parents' experiences.

Warning Signs, Identification, and Reactions to a Child's Hearing Loss

Warning Signs

Many of the minority parents reported that their first suspicions of hearing loss emanated from a home test such as pot banging or vacuuming or from suggestions of family members or caregivers. For example, one parent's babysitter suggested that the child was slow to speak. The following couple described their initial suspicions:

> *Wife: We called him, and I told him he's lookin' at the TV and I'm calling his name, when he was 2½. He didn't want to turn around.*
>
> *Husband: I got a pot, and I banged on it, and he didn't respond.*
> (Interview 2)

Another mother reported this incident:

> *Well, it was between 7 and 9 months. Umm, something dropped in my room, and I felt he should've, it should've startled him. So he was laying on my bed, and when I laid beside him and I said something in his ear, and he never responded. So that was my first, I had never ever suspected that he was hearing impaired. I always thought up until that time that he was a hearing child.* (Survey 17)

Yet another mother explained the efforts the family made to get her child's attention:

> *As far as the hearing part went, um, the only way we could get his atten-*
> *tion is if we pounded on the floor . . . and then it would gather his atten-*
> *tion, and he would turn around and look at us to see what we would want.*
> *But, uh, yeah, it, I think at 11 months, we finally said that something defi-*
> *nitely is wrong, and we went and had him checked out.* (Survey 76)

Identification

When the parents contacted their medical or audiological professionals about their suspicions of hearing loss, the actual identification of the hearing loss was sometimes delayed because the professionals told them that they were "overly worried" or "paranoid" or that reliable hearing tests could not be performed on young children. A dismissal of parents' concerns by medical professionals was common among White and minority respondents alike. Although it is not unique to minority parents, this experience is important for understanding how and why many children with a hearing loss are identified quite late. The national survey results indicate that the age at identification was significantly later for Hispanic (27.2 months) and Asian Pacific (26.8 months) children than it was for Black (20.6 months) or White (21.4 months) children. One mother described her experiences this way:

> *So I took him to the pediatrician, and he said, "No, there's nothing wrong*
> *with him. You're just a worried mom. This is your first child, and you*
> *know, you're paranoid." And I kept taking him back and kept saying the*
> *same thing, "I think something's wrong with his hearing." I would do my*
> *own little hearing tests around the house. I'd bang pots and pans togeth-*
> *er. Sometimes he would respond, and I would think, "Oh, OK, he can*
> *hear." Then other times he wouldn't respond. But anyway, I kept taking*
> *him back to the pediatrician, and finally he said, "To make you happy, I'll*
> *send you to a specialist." And he sent us to an ENT [ear, nose, and throat*
> *specialist].* (Survey 185)

The doctor found fluid in the child's ears and prescribed antibiotics. When that did not clear up the problem, they put tubes in his ears. About 2 months later, they did a brain stem hearing test and identified his profound hearing loss.

After experiencing many problems with their child in a preschool program, the following parents learned during their child's kindergarten health screening test that he had a hearing problem:

You know he had these problems along the way, and we never knew it was hearing related. Until we had him screened for kindergarten. You know they had the physical that's required for kindergarten. And at that time, they tested his hearing, and I remember the girl testing it again. And you know she came back in. You know, you want to see the results. She gave me the paper, and I said, "Oh, what does this mean?" And she said, "Oh, he hears like an old man." And I was just so stunned, like, "What do you mean?" But the referral was that we go to a hearing doctor, I mean an ear, nose, and throat doctor, who did the test again and confirmed it. So we did not find out 'til 5 years old. Well, actually he was 5½. And by the time we got to the audiologist, you know, I find out, wow, there are ways that he could have been screened much earlier. And so that, you know, you kinda kick yourself, well, why didn't I know? His pediatrician said he could hear, the speech therapist said she checked his hearing, but apparently they . . . didn't know. I mean, they, you know, my pediatrician said, well, he couldn't have tested him earlier because it wouldn't be reliable. (Survey 186)

Thus, the discovery of this child's hearing loss was delayed because the doctor dismissed the mother's concerns and because of the lack of information about reliable hearing tests that are available for infants and young children. Gerner de Garcia (1993) also reports delayed identification for Hispanic children resulting from doctors' dismissals of mothers' concerns. She suggests a number of factors to account for these dismissals, such as a lack of Spanish-speaking professionals, limited access to health care, or perceptions of the mother as incompetent. Another possible contributor to a delay is parental denial of a child's problem. Families from poor countries may not be able to verify their suspicions until they immigrate to the United States, where testing and services are more widely available.

Delayed identification means delayed intervention, resulting in slowed progress in language and speech and perhaps a loss of self-esteem (see chapter 3).

Reactions to a Child's Hearing Loss

Parents were asked about their initial reactions when they learned of their child's hearing loss. Like other hearing parents, they described feelings of shock, grief, and devastation. The following mother discussed her family's reaction as well as her own:

> *I remember my sister calling and feeling so bad for me, I mean everybody just like, you know, and when you think about it now, it's not bad, it's only hearing loss. But when you're dealing with the possibility of life-threatening illness and hearing loss, it just seems so bad. It was a really terrible weekend. I prayed so much. And you know I cried a lot. I'm sure, but, um, we got over that.* (Survey 186)

Reactions to the deaf Hispanic child by extended family members, influenced by cultural beliefs about disability, may include pity and powerful stigmas. The child may be isolated because other parents believe deafness to be contagious (Steinberg, Davila, Collazo, Loew, & Fischgrund, 1997). Inaccurate understandings equate deafness with cognitive delays and fears of lifelong dependence. Deafness may also be equated with illness and provoke a search for a miraculous cure (Ramsey, 2000).

The absence of a partner may increase the shock of identification. The NPP survey data indicate that 40% of the Black/African American and mixed-race children were living in single-parent households, compared to 15% of White children. One recently divorced mother felt very much alone at the time of the diagnosis. Religion and a supportive family helped her to adjust:

And at that point you feel kind of helpless. . . . At the time, I had got a divorce, and it was like I was a struggling parent trying to find out ways that I as a single parent could better my child. And it was really frustrating because no one would tell me nothing . . . and so we live with what God has given him. And he does just fine. And we all cope just fine with it. He's very much accepted into our family. He's not an outcast or anything like that. I think the most you can do is educate your child very well so he can function in the world and give him lots of love. (Survey 53)

Support from an extended family is echoed in another mother's response when we asked who was the most helpful to her at the time of the diagnosis:

My family. My family was, my sisters. I have like eight of them, and they were all really helpful (laughter). We cried a lot, but we started immediately trying to find programs for when he was old enough to start a program. And we didn't find one 'til he was 4 . . . 'cuz I was really trying to keep him at home. (Survey 202)

Concerns about Rights, Discrimination, Aspirations, and Financial Concerns

Rights and Discrimination

The issue of fighting for a child's rights and against discrimination emerged frequently in the interviews with this subgroup of parents. One mother spoke of being a "strong advocate" for her son. When we asked about her concerns at the time of her child's diagnosis, she commented:

My concerns? And even now [deep breath], fighting for his rights. For him to be treated equal. Umm, being accepted. Umm, I just wanted him to be treated fairly, and, uh, that about sums it up. . . . I did visit the school in [local town]. They have basketball, cheerleaders, just everything at a hearing school. I would love to see that in a school for children that are deaf. They want to be included. I would love to see that. This is pretty hard for me, seeing already discrimination with my son. . . . I would just love for him to be anything that he wants to do in the school like the hearing children. (Survey 17)

Aspirations

Parents also had concerns that their child's hearing loss might result in their not being able to accomplish their life goals. These parents' comments illustrate this theme:

I mean, even though he's only gonna be 8 years old in June, one day I would like for him to go to college. (Survey 53)

My son loves baseball. I would like him to play on a team, but not all the kids may understand the fact that my son is deaf. That means it would take more input from me to push him a little. Sometimes you may not want to push them too hard. You want him to make his own decision and things like that. How far would you push him before you push him over the edge? That type of thing. [A deaf adult friend] said he played with everybody just like a normal kid. He said push him a little and see what happens. Which is what I have to do now. Push him a little and see what happens. (Interview 2)

Financial Concerns

The NPP survey indicates that in Hispanic households, mothers often did not work outside the home (68%) or had lower-paying jobs. In African American families, the mother was more often working (51%), with about one third in clerical positions and another third in lower-skill-level jobs. These employment conditions contribute to the challenges that minority parents face with deaf and hard of hearing children. One mother described her frustration in getting Social Security coverage for deafness-related expenses:

Right now, I'm still trying to get his Social Security thing going. . . . It has been difficult because they're not making it easy. I know a lot of people who've gotten Social Security for lesser things. It's not like he's faking his hearing loss and stuff like that. I'm still in the process of that. That has been very difficult. (Interview 2)

Another mother felt her child needed more speech therapy than the school provided. Because her insurance did not cover the expense, extra therapy created an economic hardship:

They felt like he was getting it at school. We didn't feel like it was enough. . . . They give it to you at school, but they only give you like 30 minutes a week. (Survey 334)

Other parents expressed frustration with insurance companies' high deductible fees. Because of the lower economic status of many minority families, financial expenditures are a special concern.

Because no services for deaf children were available close to their home, one family sent their son to a residential school many miles away. The mother wanted to be involved in her son's education and to support the school when behavior problems arose. However, she found the distance created a financial burden for her:

If my son gets in trouble or something, they want me to drive 150 miles, 300 miles to come get him. And that's so hard on you. And, um, here it is, I'm barely making it, and I'm a struggling mother and they want me to, I mean, I know this is my kid and this is coming out wrong, but you gotta understand the background behind it. If you're poor, and they want you to come get your kid, you don't have the gas, your car barely runs, and I don't think that they see that. But yet there's nothing I can do because there's nothing up here for him so I can put him close to me. (Survey 53)

Gerner de Garcia (2000) reports that Hispanic families may be unable to obtain services or participate in their child's center-based program because of lack of transportation or child care, work schedules, or cultural or language barriers. With this knowledge in mind, the NPP invitation to participate in focus groups included reimbursement for transportation, child care, food, and financial incentives.

Support: Family/Siblings, Religion, and Professionals

Interviewed parents reported varying degrees of support from their family, the child's siblings, their religion, and the professionals they encountered in their child's early years. Some extended family members felt sorry for them; others provided active support and acceptance.

Support from Family/Siblings

Previous studies of these groups document the importance of and support from extended family members in Hispanic, African American, and Asian families (Cheng, 2000; Mapp & Hudson, 1997; Rodriguez & Santiviago, 1991). In the NPP survey, both White and Black families generally reported strong support from their extended families, whereas Hispanic families reported their relatives to be less supportive.

Despite the importance of extended family in many cultural groups, not all of the minority families with deaf children receive support from their extended family. No Hispanic parent in the study by Steinberg et al. (1997) received help from their extended families. However, five of nine participants had relocated from Puerto Rico in order to obtain services for the deaf child. (This was also true of a participant in one of our focus groups.) NPP parents reported making many sacrifices and significant life changes for their children. Four families moved from other countries or across state lines to improve opportunities for their children.

One supportive grandmother heard about cochlear implants in her work at a pediatric hospital:

She saw a sign saying "cochlear implant patients" or something. So she called the hospital the next day and made an appointment . . . and 3

days later we were at the appointment getting him evaluated, and with-
in I guess a month or so he had qualified as a candidate [and he was
implanted 6 months later]. (Survey 185)

In some families, the siblings were very supportive, and in others they had not adjusted to their deaf or hard of hearing brother or sister. As sometimes happens, the following younger brother wanted to be like his older deaf sibling:

He's got a younger brother . . . (who) is very close. He's 2 years old, and
that little guy is learning sign language. He switches between sign lan-
guage and speaking because he sees Mommy do the sign language and
Brother do the sign language, and he wants to do everything big brother
does. (Interview)

Some siblings refused to use sign language. In the following family, the older sister was very embarrassed by her hard of hearing brother's hearing aids:

I don't know, we're very accepting of glasses, you know, but hearing aids
is just another thing. And my daughter was so devastated, too, and she
was so embarrassed of him, wearing hearing aids, she hated the hearing
aids. She would say this in front of him. (Survey 186)

When this child's hearing loss was identified, the mother sought books to explain this to her hearing children. She found several about profoundly deaf children but none about hard of hearing children. She plans to write books for siblings of hard of hearing children when she retires.

Support from Religion

In the NPP survey, Black (59%) and Hispanic (45%) families reported that their religion was very helpful in terms of support, as compared to White

families (28%). In one family, the parents, grandmother, and uncle are taking sign language classes. In this family, the grandfather is a minister, and
they reported the following:

> *Wife: Prayers help a lot, too.*

> *Husband: You can't stop believing, like you're saying. You got to have your
> beliefs.* (Interview)

Another mother explained that it was prayer that got them through the
initial shock. She said that their support came from "prayer, friends, um,
reading the Word, getting on our knees" (Survey 334).

Rodriguez and Santiviago (1991), Ramsey (2000), and Steinberg and
colleagues (1997) also report a strong link between religion and beliefs
about disabilities. In the study by Steinberg et al., the Hispanic families
made reference to God as the cause of their child's deafness. However, that
study made no mention of religion as a source of support. Mapp and
Hudson (1997) report that African American and Hispanic families who
experienced fewer adjustment problems and lower levels of stress also
reported more frequent church attendance. These parents indicated that
their religion was a helpful source of support.

Support from Professionals

The degree of support from professionals varied considerably among the
interviewed parents. A husband and wife who were interviewed described
their family's meeting with doctors at the hospital after their child's hearing loss was identified. The mother, father, child, grandmother, grandfather,
uncle, and godmother all attended. They went to learn more about the
child's deafness, the causative factors, the tests that were used, and the management of hearing aids, asking questions and discussing their concerns:

> *They explain to you how they put the hearing aids on and the volume of
> the hearing aids. [A staff member] was speaking Spanish to my mother
> because she didn't understand English. So she was translating everything*

that [the doctor] had to say in Spanish. They had a meeting there to teach them what was the reason he was deaf, his hearing aids, how to put them on. (Interview)

The following family described the friendship and personal concern of these professionals, whom they still see occasionally:

Like anybody in general, there are certain things you want to hear and certain things you don't want to hear. When they told us that he had a hearing loss, it was kind of hard to accept at first, but they directed us in the right way of going about and getting his hearing aids and so on. To this day they are still helping us. (Interview)

Although this family received extraordinary, positive support from professionals, this is not always the case for minority families. Lack of fluency in the family's language, underrepresentation of ethnic groups in the professional community, or cultural insensitivity can lead to less positive experiences (Gerner de Garcia, 2000; Wathum–Ocama, 2000). A contrasting experience is evident in the comments of another mother, whose doctor told her that her child had significant medical problems and would need special services and that the child should be in an early intervention program getting physical therapy. Even though she was living in a major metropolitan area, the doctor was not able to give her any referrals. She moved to another state in search of services for her daughter and found an early intervention program that agreed to do the evaluation free of charge:

Yeah, they were just, like I said, so supportive, and they always looked for the positive about what she could do, and their whole philosophy was to build off of what they could do and would try to add to that. The medical profession is always focused on what they can't do and what the problem is. (Survey 075)

Another parent described a positive relationship with the audiologist who helped her understand her child's hearing loss by explaining what he could and could not hear and how to help him adjust to his hearing aids:

Like I didn't . . . even understand that . . . it was the consonants he couldn't hear. You know, and she explained to me, like, what sounds and gave me a chart with . . . letters. And then it all made sense. Oh, no wonder he always drops his "s's" and never says "s's," and, you know, I mean, the audiologist probably provided me with the most information. (Survey 186)

Most of the parents were able to describe an educator who was very supportive, either in the early intervention program or in school:

There was a girl who was his teacher, and we became personal friends, and she gave inside tips to things that nobody would tell us . . . and it's kind of like she opened my eyes to things, and she told me how I need to go around the system to get the most for my child. (Survey 53)

Parents also described the support they received from educational professionals for disciplining their child. One mother who felt guilty for punishing her daughter before her hearing loss was identified explained:

We found different ways of dealing with her behaviors because we understood why she was doing it. But everyone kind of helped me adjust to the change. So, like I said, not punishing her but working with her. . . . Everybody was just (helpful), the school personnel. (Survey 111)

Communication at Home and School

Mapp and Hudson (1997) investigated the relationship between African American and Hispanic parents' stress levels, their children's behavior problems, and their children's signing skills. Parents of children with good signing skills reported both less stress and fewer behavior problems. Steinberg and her colleagues (1997) also report that minority parents perceive that their children experience behavioral difficulties that they attribute to unsatisfactory communication between the child and family. Issues of access to services, severity of hearing loss, finances, family values, and extent of knowledge of various options all influence communication choices (see chapter 2).

Parents expressed concerns about their ability to sign and communicate with their deaf children. One parent described using only home gestures before their son started school:

We just speak with each other. We don't sign. . . . We probably gesture, but still I would like to speak to him. I don't like to sign. . . . I'll probably never sign. . . . I want to speak to him. [His wife is learning to sign because their son signs at school.] (Focus Group 3)

Ramsey (2000) reports that Mexican-heritage mothers tried to sign whereas the fathers only spoke Spanish. Often their extended families criticized them because they did not teach their deaf child to speak Spanish. In one NPP family, the father recognized that the child, exposed to sign at school, would likely surpass the parents' skills. A mother recognized her own lack of signing skills as a problem:

And sometimes it is frustrating dealing with them. 'Cuz you have to deal with them different than you deal with the hearing child. There's things you cannot talk about to them 'cuz you don't know the signs for it, and you're afraid you're going to miscommunicate. (Survey 202)

Steinberg and colleagues (1997) report mixed communication abilities in Hispanic families. Many families attended sign classes, used signs sporadically at home, and believed that the deaf child really could hear and understand. Regardless of whether these responses reflect parental denial or lack of information about deafness, they have serious consequences for communication and language development. Communication becomes more complex when the home language is not English and the family, child, and service providers must deal with trilingual challenges (Cheng, 2000; Gerner de Garcia, 2000).

Two minority families chose a cochlear implant for their child. In chapter 5 one of these describes their excitement when the child responded to his name after the surgery. The other family was frustrated and disappointed when the expected speech progress did not occur:

> And, uh, it was probably 3 years after . . . he was implanted that I did find out that he should have been having a regular conversation and speech at 18 months postimplant, which he just still wasn't doing, and he is still not doing. So we ended up going back to sign language for him and teaching him sign language again. (Survey 76)

This family's experience suggests a possible lack of support for the expensive and time-consuming follow-up needed after an implant procedure, an issue that is discussed further in chapter 6.

Access to and Satisfaction with Services

Minority families reported significantly greater dissatisfaction with their medical and audiological services compared to White, non-Hispanic families. Like other survey participants, minority parents based their feelings of satisfaction with professionals on their responsiveness to the family's most pressing concerns. Interviewed parents described satisfaction with those who involved the entire family and helped them understand the meaning of their child's hearing loss. Others expressed frustration because of delay in testing due to a doctor's dismissal of their concerns or the mistaken idea that testing a young child was not possible. One mother was upset because one professional made negative comments about hearing aids to her son.

Inaccessibility of services was an issue that a number of parents mentioned. One family's options were limited because the father served in the armed forces:

We're military, so this definitely would not be the town that I'd settle in for my son. I just don't feel like he has a chance here. I visited the school for the deaf, and I felt like he was too young to be 2½ hours away from me. And I want him here, here, you know? The teacher, she's nice, but as far as services and activities, they don't have them here for hearing impaired. (Survey 17)

Other families chose to send their young children to a residential program because they did not have access to an appropriate educational setting close to home. The following mother described the emotional difficulty of having her young child so far away:

God, that's still so hard because it's still so far away. You know, they can't make me feel welcomed or involved because it's so far away. I just feel like I'm a total outcast. Everyone down there is so proficient at signing, and here I am, I'm very far away. I'm still going to school to try to better myself. And when I go down there I still don't feel comfortable 'cuz everyone signs so good. (Survey 53)

Conflicts arose within extended families related to sending a child away from home to a residential school. Ramsey (2000) reports that extended families severely criticized Mexican-heritage parents who sent their child to a distant residential program. This conflicted with a cultural belief that parents should socialize the child in their culture and language at home. Sending a child away is viewed as a sign of incompetence and a serious indictment of the parents' childrearing values.

Distance and economic hardship may also limit a family's access to sign language classes as well as its ability to participate in the child's education. This mother commented:

Because I lived so far, I didn't get away, but they offered sign language classes twice a week. And I coulda went up for it, but because I had to work, because I'm a single parent, I didn't get to go for it. (Survey 202)

Her child has recently returned home because there is a trial program in her area for 1 year. A sign language teacher comes to the home to teach the whole family. The mother thinks this is wonderful but doesn't know whether it will continue.

Parents described a high level of satisfaction with early childhood programs that sent someone to their homes to teach them sign language and other skills related to raising a child with a hearing loss. In fact, all of the parents in our largest focus group received home visits of this kind. This in-home support contributed to the praise and appreciation parents expressed for the teachers and professionals working at their children's school. One mother commented:

> *And they sent a person out to talk to me, you know, about the educational ways they can go at his young age. . . . And that lady, she was a godsend. She worked miracles with me and my son [laughter]. And she started telling me, you know, how to first start off signing, you know, one-word signs, getting him to recognize 'em and all that. And they come into my home so, you know, I didn't have to make schedules to go to [city name] or nothing like that. Their coming into my home helped me a lot.* (Survey 98)

Several parents mentioned their feelings of isolation because they did not have access to a parent support group. Two parents with hard of hearing children were unable to find a parent support group because these were organized only for parents of deaf children:

> *You know what I didn't have is other parents to talk to. You know, and I was just really kinda going it alone.* (Survey 186)

Other parents did not participate in a support group because they were unaware of their availability or the services offered were too far away or meetings conflicted with other family responsibilities.

Educational Services

Concerns about education may overlap with satisfaction with educational services. One parent felt she was forced to accept a placement in a public school for her child. When she observed a hearing school where the deaf children were all in one self-contained classroom, her reaction was the following:

I . . . checked out their program that they had offered, and at the end of it, I was very, very discouraged. Very. And I told our head of education up here that I did not want my child mainstreamed. I wanted him to be in a hearing impaired school because he is hearing impaired. They can deal with him more there, and he can learn more what he needs instead of the environment they have up here. And he kept sayin' "Well, you know, they have to be, they need to be introduced to hearing children, also." And I said, "I know that." I said, "My child—the only time he's around other hearing impaired children is at school." I said, "Around here it's all hearing people." And, uh, when I had checked out the [mainstreamed] school, they had had like ages of 6 to 11 in one class [setting], you know, all that different age groups in one class with one teacher. If they went down the hallways, say they got disoriented and lost their way back to their room, the other teachers—they're not certified in any kinda signin.' They don't know sign, and they wouldn't know what my child was sayin.' And at the pep rallies and school activities, none of it was signed. The kids were just sittin' there, they didn't really know what was goin' on. They were just watchin' the other reactions of the people around 'em. Nothin' was signed to 'em so they could understand what the pep rally was for or anything like that, and I was really discouraged . . . and I got out of there. (Survey 98)

Other parents whose children went to public schools expressed satisfaction when the staff provided them with information and a positive attitude about their child's potential. One mother illustrated the importance of professionals' willingness to listen:

*They were just always willing to listen, and they went through every-
thing. So they started her in the services. But they were always willing to
listen to any of my concerns, and they were always so tuned in. They just
so firmly believe that parents know their children best. And that those are
the people who they need to support and to listen to and follow through
on the concerns that they had.* (Survey 75)

Some parents whose child went to a school for deaf children expressed
satisfaction because the staff provided them with information about
devices such as doorbells and alarm clocks designed for deaf people. This
mother described her general satisfaction with her son's residential school
experience:

*Well, they basically get him ready to deal with the world, you know. They
have lipreading, sign language, speech, and I mean it just made him feel
like he was part of everything. He didn't feel left out. And I mean, I don't
know, they had a wonderful program. The only thing bad about it, he had
to be away from home all week. He could only come home on the weekends.* (Survey 202)

Parents perceived Individualized Educational Plan (IEP) meetings both
positively and negatively. Some parents described the venue of their IEP
meetings with the professionals as an adversarial setting in which they had
to fight for their child's rights. One mother commented:

*I'm finding that there is a struggle with everything, fighting for his rights.
Umm, he has an IEP coming up, and I've been told that I'm probably really gonna have to have a battle because I want an interpreter 'cuz this . . .
soccer is through the school. So I want an interpreter. I want the school to
provide an interpreter. So it's pretty tough here.* (Survey 17)

Another mother has a positive recollection of her experiences in an IEP
meeting:

And you know, we have IEP meetings every year, and that's when we—I go down to the school and we sit around . . . what [child] accomplished this year, what he needs to be accomplishin,' what else, you know, do I see anything that my son needs more of, and anything that I need or if I have any questions. The school's really great with me. (Survey 98)

Differences in satisfaction relate to differences in support, access to services, and the parents' frame of reference.

Conclusion

The views of the minority parents we report here are enlightening in terms of the effectiveness of services and the supportiveness of professionals. Although generalizations or stereotyping based on race or ethnicity are detrimental, it is useful to note the issues documented here in order to assist minority families more effectively. As the population of the United States continues to boom and the schools serving deaf and hard of hearing children become more diverse, it is vital that these issues be addressed.

Among the significant issues that call for further study are the following: (1) lower levels of satisfaction with services that minority parents report, (2) cultural and language influences on communication choices and educational placements, and (3) access to services that encourage the involvement and support of minority parents. Studies of the reasons for the changing demographics might provide insights into this subgroup's future need for services. In addition, conducting research in Spanish with Spanish-speaking parents is important in order to obtain information from those parents who were excluded from this study because of its use of English only. Comparative research between minority and White families might also shed light on the concerns or problems that minority members face and ways in which the addition of a deaf or hard of hearing child might compound them. Finally, comparisons with Spanish-speaking families with and without children who are deaf or hard of hearing could illuminate difficulties that these families face while participating in their children's schooling.

Cultural sensitivity is of the utmost importance. Professionals need to understand that every situation is unique and that parents' educational levels, marital and employment status, housing situations, and location influence people from all cultures. Affluence and access to services have always been powerfully linked, and we need to consider ways to make services available to all families, especially for those who cope with economic challenges. To serve the needs of deaf and hard of hearing children, professionals need to address these issues. No child should experience delayed identification of hearing loss, but late identification is even more unacceptable if it results from the dismissal—because of a parent's minority status—of such concerns. Further study of the needs of minority deaf and hard of hearing children should be a priority.

Chapter 8

Parent to Parent: Do What's Best for Your Child

Never give up hope. Their kids are bright. . . . Most importantly is patience, love, communication with understanding at an early age. (Survey 71)

And if you stand beside your kids and teach 'em, they will do it, and it takes a lot of patience. I don't need to tell you, you know—having deaf children. But patience is like one of the key issues that you have to have. Just have patience with your kids and teach them everything. And, really, when your children stop and don't understand what's going on, just try to explain to them what is going on. If you don't have the language for it, just do the best you can. (Focus Group 2)

Always maintain your sense of humor. It helps. Just remember that you are the parent. And you will always know your child better than anyone else. And to remember that decisions you make can be changed; they're not locked in stone. (Survey 257)

In this chapter parents of deaf and hard of hearing children share their advice with parents who have recently discovered that their child has a hearing loss. Previous studies point to such advice from other parents as the most pressing need at the time a child's hearing loss is identified. Parents indicated that what they most wanted at that moment was to be able to talk with other parents with a similar child (Luterman & Kurtzer-White, 1999; Tolland, 1995). Parents who have lived through the uncertainty and frustration of decision making have tremendous experience and expertise to share. The format for parents interacting with each other can vary, ranging from formally designed parent support groups to Internet communications. The effects of contacts with other parents also vary, ranging from increased knowledge of options to decreased stress in the familial relationship (Hintermair, 2000b; Singer et al., 1999).

The advice in this chapter is based on the interviews with the full range of parents in the phone survey and focus groups, as well as comments parents made at a session that the authors conducted at the July 2000 meeting of the American Society for Deaf Children (Meadow-Orlans, Sass-Lehrer, & Mertens, 2000). When we asked parents to advise other parents who had recently discovered that their child was deaf or hard of hearing, a number of interesting themes emerged. Overwhelmingly the parents emphasized that each child is an individual and families must make decisions that are appropriate for the unique child and family:

> *They can decide what fits best for them and their family and their situation. I think it's different for every child.* (Survey 75)

They also stressed that it is important to see the child first and to love the child:

> *Tell them he is still a normal child and give lots of love and learn how to communicate as soon as possible.* (Survey 29)

> *See their child as a child first and not the disability. If we know that something isn't working the way it should, sometimes we focus on the thing that isn't working the way it should and lose sight of the other. . . . I guess it's to keep the perspective to looking at all the positive the child does have, you know, and focus on the person first and then his needs second.* (Survey 242)

They advised treating the child as normally as possible and not ignoring the aspects of childhood that are important for all children, hearing or deaf:

> *Sometimes the hearing impaired child—that becomes their identity. "Oh, they're hearing impaired," rather than, "This is a person who has a hear-*

ing problem." That helped me. I would not let the hearing impairment define her. And so then I could let her do all kinds of normal things 'cause she was Shatasha first and Shatasha had to do these things. . . . My child has played T-ball with an all-hearing team. She has played soccer with an all-hearing team. One soccer team, all the kids, the mothers were taking it upon themselves to buy books on sign language so they could communicate with her. That was tremendous. I couldn't believe it. (Survey 242)

In addition to the overall sentiment that deaf and hard of hearing children are children first and deserve normal childhood experiences, other themes that emerged include the importance of acknowledging feelings and moving on, seeking support from other parents, becoming knowledgeable about options and resources, advocating for an appropriate education, and fostering the child's self-esteem. These five themes form the basis of the remainder of this chapter.

Acknowledge Your Feelings and Move On

It is not uncommon for hearing parents to feel a sense of loss when they discover that their child is deaf or hard of hearing. Elsewhere in this book, reactions to the identification of a hearing loss have been detailed. Here, parents reflect on the need to get past the stage of shock and grieving:

I guess the first thing I would do is just comfort them because, you know, it's a grieving process because it's like "my child will never hear." You know, it's like some part of them has died. So I would just comfort them, and then I'd reassure them that there are other people out there. There are other parents. I would try to encourage them to grieve but get over it and just try to go on. . . . Just do what's best for your child. Don't sit there and let your child just not have any services. You have to think about the child first. (Survey 317)

To probably look at grief therapy and realize that the reason that a lot of things are falling apart around their ankles is because of grief. And the

anger is because of grief and to expect the grief and work with it accord-
ingly, because it can be pretty consuming. (Survey 348)

I would say that when you get a piece of bad news, there's no way to feel
right at that moment except bad. And you just have to get over it, let the
bad feeling pass. You have to mourn for the loss for what you thought was
gonna be this child. But the child himself hasn't changed a bit from the
way he was born. You just didn't know these things about him. But he is
still an interesting, contributing, fascinating person who has a place in the
world. And he'll reach his potential with just the extra help that he needs.
(Survey 121)

Well, going back to the beginning, of course, I was devastated. I cried.
You just have that. You grieve because you're losing all your ideals. But
you know, when you have a child, you have all these ideas that your
child's gonna do this. You know, basically, they're gonna go to kinder-
garten, play sports, do this, do that, whatever, and gonna be smart. You
just have all these thoughts, all these plans. You get hit by this and it's like,
"Man, everything's gone." You have no future in your mind for your child
any more. You don't know. But you kinda have to get past all that . . .
because it doesn't do you or your child any good to just mope about it.
(Survey 251)

I see a lot of parents just kinda standin' there waiting for somebody to
take the ball, and I think professionals know when parents are involved
early that they can make a big difference. And I don't think parents—
they're so locked into their grief, and somebody just needs to, like, slap
'em and say, "OK, this is not what you had intended, but if you don't get
involved and get involved quickly, then your child's gonna suffer."
(Survey 293)

A common theme throughout these parents' comments is the importance of acknowledging feelings at the time of the diagnosis. If one views
the discovery of a hearing loss from the perspective of the loss of the

hoped-for child, then a normal part of the reaction may be a period of grieving. However, parents also suggest that getting past the grieving is in the child's best interest. If parents continue to let their feelings paralyze them, the child will suffer. NPP survey results suggest that the majority of parents have accepted the hearing loss by the time the child is 6 or 7 years old. With the implementation of universal hearing screening at birth it is possible that parents will accept the hearing loss earlier in their child's life. It may not be the age of identification but rather the provision of early intervention services and support for families that appears to help parents resolve their feelings of grief and move on. The study by Pipp-Siegel, Blair, Deas, Pressman, and Yoshinaga-Itano (1999) looks at the emotional availability of mothers with 42 children, half of whom were D/HH and half, hearing (20–27 months and 15–21 months respectively). They find no difference in emotional availability of mothers and increased levels of maternal sensitivity to their children when they receive early intervention services and are satisfied with their social support. Pipp-Siegel et al. suggest that early intervention is an important factor. Yoshinaga-Itano and her colleagues state that families experience less stress and faster resolution of grief when hearing loss is identified early and accompanied by appropriate early intervention services (Yoshinaga-Itano & Marion Downs Center for Infant Hearing, 2001).

Many of the deaf parents in this study did not express feelings of shock or grieving on learning about their child's hearing loss. Indeed, most of them indicated feeling acceptance and sometimes happiness because the child is like them. Nevertheless, some deaf parents commented that they experienced concerns with the birth of their deaf child because they knew the challenges they themselves had faced growing up. One deaf parent described the reactions of other deaf parents who found out their child was deaf:

They were so happy or thrilled. Sometimes I do see some deaf parents might be disappointed in knowing their children are deaf knowing there [are] limited services or accessibility, but once again emphasizing . . . that in the past 50 years there were barely none available for the deaf. But with today's technology and more awareness and more exposure [to] inform them, their child [will] have better benefits and chances than what they went through. Talk with deaf parents who raised deaf children. Smile. (Survey 376)

Research generally supports a positive family life in homes with deaf parents and deaf children (Meadow-Orlans, 2002a). Parent and child share a defining characteristic enabling them to share cultural experiences.

The final thought in this thematic section relates to moving on once parents have recognized their feelings, and then taking responsibility for their child:

In general, it doesn't matter if you've got a deaf kid or not. I think that ulti-mately we really have to be responsible for our kids. We can't just let social services always seek us out. We have to be willing and be receptive and do what we have to do. I think that's part of it, too. I know that, if I had just let it go, I probably would not have been as fortunate to be hooked into everything that I did find out about. If I just kind of sat back waiting for people to come to me. You know, parents have to take that responsi-bility. (Survey 61)

The process of moving on and finding direction for action can come from other parents. The next section explores advice concerning contact with other parents.

Seek Support from Other Parents

NPP survey results show that parents view contact with other parents as helpful. Ninety percent of the parents in the study indicated that other parents were a helpful source of support, whether it was provided by a for-mal parent support group or informal contact with other parents. Parent support groups were one way to facilitate dealing with the initial shock, but they were also seen as an ongoing, valuable resource. Many comments illustrate the importance of parent support groups:

I think it's important to go through that [grieving process] and have support with that. You know, find somebody who has either been through it or understands what that's like and kind of lets you go through that. (Survey 80)

Anyone who's hearing and has a deaf child, get involved in a parent support group 'cause I thought it was very beneficial. I mean, I wasn't one who was a real baby person when I was growing up, and I started having my family very late. So I just recommend that to anyone. You meet lots of other mothers that way. (Survey 260)

Getting together with other parents, too. You know, we got to know them, which was helpful, too, 'cuz we all have the same thing in common, so that was real nice. Getting some support there. (Survey 21)

If you've never been around the Deaf community or anything, you don't really know what's going on. . . . There are people, there's like the support groups, the parent groups and that, that you kinda go with. And you know, it helps to go to a parent group even though you don't want to talk about your problems or whatever. Somebody there is gonna feel that same way you do. And it will help you. (Survey 251)

Hintermair (2000a) studied the relationship between the amount of contact with other parents of deaf and hard of hearing children and the parents' stress levels in Germany. He reported that parents who frequently met with other parents of deaf and hard of hearing children reported less isolation, stronger emotional bonds with their child, and greater acceptance of the child. Through sharing experiences, the parents were able to develop a better understanding of their situation and gain new perspectives. Parents also emphasized the benefits of giving mutual practical help in coping with everyday challenges. American mothers reported similar results. Those with more social support were better adjusted personally to their deaf or hard of hearing child (Calderon & Greenberg, 1999).

Several parents indicated that it was difficult to find someone to talk to, either because their child's hearing loss was different from those of others around them or because of factors such as geographic isolation or the presence of an additional condition. They commented both on their frustration and on ways they found to connect with other parents:

Just encourage them to join, because I never did, and I think it would've helped, and it would've been nice to have had somebody else to talk to besides the teacher or an itinerant or something like that. It would have been nice to have another parent, a shoulder to lean on once in a while. And I would just like to be there. In fact, I've tried to contact people about doing that. You know, give 'em my name and, you know, that I'm willing to talk to people. But it's never worked out. (Survey 317)

If they can, talk to others. I didn't have that here. I didn't have anybody, you know. Because high-frequency hearing losses probably aren't that common. (Survey 186)

My sons had progressive losses, and they are now 13 and 9 years old. We were looking for support, but everyone there had their kids identified at birth. I couldn't really find that. They didn't seem interested in talking to me. Our kids don't fit in because they speak well. SHHH [Self-Help for Hard of Hearing People] shuns sign language, but sign language has been positive for our children. We don't have that Deaf community. They go to summer camps, but they don't have friends like them. We expose them more and more to sign language. It is hard to find support and finding someone with a similar situation. (Parent comment, American Society for Deaf Children Conference, July 2000)

Some parents solved the problem of finding other parents to talk to by going through agencies or using Internet technology:

Seek out an agency that could put you in touch with other hearing parents of deaf children. Don't isolate yourself or try not to let the situation isolate you or make you feel as though no one understands. Having a net-work or having a resource where hearing parents of deaf children could be paired with another hearing parent of a deaf child so that they would have somebody to kind of, you know . . . bat ideas around or, you know, form a friendship. That's what I did with a young girl whose child was diagnosed, and we're several years apart in age, but we have remained very, very close, and her little boy is the same age as mine. And just net-working and doing things with her. (Survey 348)

We found a lot of support through the Internet. We can find similar families with the same issues and helpful information. Parent chat groups provide real information. The Internet is a fabulous tool for sup-port. (Parent comment, American Society for Deaf Children Con-ference, July 2000)

Mothers often assume more child care responsibilities than fathers, especially when the children are deaf (Meadow-Orlans & Sass-Lehrer, 1995). Fathers of deaf or hard of hearing children are less likely than their wives to learn to sign and to attend parent meetings. Spousal support can be a source of strong positive reassurance or increased anxiety, depending on the spouse's reaction to the hearing loss. Calderon and Low (1998) report that language and academic-related test scores of children in homes with the father present were significantly higher than in homes where fathers were absent. One father described his emotional state as follows:

When we went into the school, the father wants to feel in control, and someone besides him knows a better way. The father's esteem is stomped. The medical industry squashes that self-confidence. You have to put your confidence in another person. The father is in the back seat. Many others feel the same way, and it's like your child is someone else's. It forces you to trust other people, and that's why you don't see fathers as involved. (Parent comment, American Society for Deaf Children Conference, July 2000)

Several mothers suggested that their husbands had a more difficult time adjusting to the identification of a hearing loss than they did:

I don't know if it's true for everyone, but my husband took a lot longer to get through the denial phase than I did. Hang in there, because you are supporting your spouse, too. And don't argue or fight with him, just listen to their feelings and explain that things aren't the way we want them to be. But they're the way they are, and try to listen. Because I know my husband took a long time to [get] over the initial shock and hurt of having a hearing impaired child. Start reading everything that you can get your hands on because it can ruin your marriage. . . . You are now at a high risk for divorce because you have a child with a disability, especially hearing impairment. . . . It's really important to keep talking to your spouse and try to look in the same direction. (Survey 286)

One father who admitted to being frightened and angry at first commented:

It's surprising how many wonderful people you are going to find out there. All of those people are doing this because they love helping the children. I am so thankful for those people helping my wife early on. Without those people I don't know where we'd be. (Parent comment, American Society for Deaf Children Conference, July 2000)

Both mothers and fathers recognized that their spouses' reactions might be different from their own. One spouse may have to carry the load alone for a while if the other needs more time to adjust. Children with disabilities can either increase marital stress (Brand & Coetzer, 1994) or strengthen family ties (Koester & Meadow-Orlans, 1990). Many parents emphasized the importance of recognizing the differences in feelings and providing mutual support.

Become Knowledgeable about Resources and Options

Parents emphasized the importance of learning as much as possible about resources and options for meeting the needs of their children, as well as advocating for appropriate services. Parents also emphasized the importance of educating themselves about tests that are appropriate for infants and young children even before the identification of hearing loss. They felt it was necessary to have that knowledge in order to ascertain appropriate testing early in their child's life, especially if the medical professionals dismissed their suspicions of a hearing loss. This includes learning about the options for communication and education. They recommended a wide variety of resources including associations that serve various deaf and hard of hearing constituencies, such as Self-Help for Hard of Hearing People, A. G. Bell, and the American Society for Deaf Children (ASDC). Appendix D provides a detailed list of resources that includes the contact information for such associations. Parents made the following comments:

People who suspect something is wrong, keep pushing the doctors. Argue, do what you have to do. . . . I really wish we had gotten that test 6 months earlier, when we first asked. (Survey 372)

I think they need to make it a point to really educate themselves. Just find out as much information as they can, talk to as many people as they can, read as much as they can. (Survey 297)

It's really important for you to find out as much, to, like, educate yourself and find out as much as you can about all the different options out there. Not feel like people tell you what they're going to do with your child. I think it's important for you to feel like you read all you can read and you've talked to everyone you can talk to, and you go to every single piece of educational thing you can go to. And so you have some sort of, like, control or power in the situation, more than if you just let people boss you around. (Survey 80)

The importance of the choice of communication mode is discussed in chapter 2. Because this is such an important issue, it is not surprising that many parents commented on learning more about the options and resources related to this choice. They frequently advised looking broadly at the options and choosing the one that is best for the child:

> *Give different options of communication modes with facts. Some kids can do well in mainstreaming school versus others who cannot do well. . . . I always believe in giving facts of different communication modes. And the most important thing for parents to know is what is the best interest for the child, not for themselves. . . . It is important to know what their child needs. It is really important to know the child's best interests, not the parents' best interests.* (Survey 376)

> *For hearing parents who find their children have a hearing loss, I would recommend that they take Deaf culture, Deaf studies, and also contact SHHH as well as NAD [National Association of the Deaf] and local schools so they can get all the information. . . . So be sure to share all facts, pros and cons.* (Survey 376)

Both hearing and deaf parents recommended consulting members of the Deaf community for advice on options and resources. As a mother of a deaf child, Tolland (1995) chose to maximize both signing and oral communication. She reports the challenges involved in learning sign language as a hearing adult and describes the help she received from the Deaf community in learning signs and teaching them to her child. Hintermair's (2000b) research with German parents indicates their stress levels were lower when they had more contact with deaf adults. These parents reported that their contact with deaf adults enhanced their ability to use effective coping strategies with their children.

Communication choices can be very complex. What one might perceive as the warring camps of sign language and oralist supporters complicates the gathering of information and considering of options for communication decisions (Tolland, 1995; Steinberg et al., 2000).

Many interviewees emphasized the importance of keeping communication open between parents and child. Even with the complexities of alternative communication modes or assistive listening devices, these interviewees counseled parents to choose a method and/or device that will allow them to communicate effectively with their child. They discussed the importance of learning sign language and of obtaining appropriate hearing aids and speech therapy. Many parents recommended the use of sign language; some expressly recommended American Sign Language. Others felt that the situation can be confusing and that it will take time to figure out what will be appropriate for the child:

I think they're so overwhelmed with all the information they're given. And they're told all of the different options, you know, there is the oral, there's the Total Communication, the manual only, there's the SEE II, and I think it's pretty overwhelming. I think it's really difficult for them to make a decision. I think most of them just decide on whatever is easiest for their family, which probably is the best decision although, I mean, for the family, but maybe not for the deaf child necessarily. But for many of them, they don't know sign language to begin with, and then signing is not really that easy for everybody to learn. I've taught many sign classes myself, and I can see some people pick it up really quickly and other people just struggle with it and give up. . . . I always tell people that they don't always have an opportunity to become proficient in sign because they don't know a lot of deaf adults. (Survey 260)

Advocate for an Appropriate Education

Several parents noted the importance of being active in a child's educational experience and accepting the responsibility of acting on their children's behalf:

I guess I think that once you've made a decision as to what you're going to do, it's not gonna do it itself. You can't, no matter what the choice is, you can't just rely on the school to do it for you because 1 hour a week, 2 hours a week, wherever the kids go, even if they're in a daily program, that's just a small portion of their life. And it's really the family that has to keep helping the child. You know, for them to really get to work. (Survey 226)

Many parents advised other parents to go to their child's school and see what is happening with the youngster. Parents are in a better position to advocate for their child if they know what is going on in the school setting:

I guess just to be sure and work with [the professionals] and, you know, get involved . . . even if it is sitting in on some of the classrooms, if they let you do that, which they did let us do. Keep in contact with them and with your child. (Survey 21)

Each family's different according to time and their views on education. It's up to each individual parent—just go see what's going on. Just sit there and watch. Go to the other classrooms and sit there and see what's gonna happen in the future. I don't have a lot of time where I can involve myself in volunteering over there. . . . Just don't be ignorant of what's going on in the child's life. Just keep the communication open between the teachers and the families. (Survey 24)

Check out the school really well. Go to the supervisor. I had second thoughts about [her son's school] because the first time he was enrolled, I went in and the first thing they did was sent me to the nurse 'cuz she has to know if he's on medication or if he has any health problems and all of this. And they just weren't very concerned, ya know, it was like OK. And I'm like "OK, well, where do I take him from here?" And they're, like, "Take him to his class," and I'm like, "OK, I don't even know where his class is." You know? Just really check the school out and tour it very well and see who you are dealing with. (Survey 24)

Parents expressed strong sentiments regarding the importance of advocating for a child:

If you're not happy with a particular school and you want to move into another one, go ahead and fight because you can fight for your child's education to get the best education possible. (Survey 163)

Be your child's best advocate is my advice. Stand up for your child, and make sure you know everything that's going on, and spend a full day at the school. You know, to know what they do every minute of every day. So you know their schedule because basically that's where I kind of got lost. I didn't know what she was doing at school. . . . So it would be to be their best advocates, stand up for them. Know your options. Ask a lot of questions; that would be my advice. (Survey 149)

I talk a lot, and I've learned over the years to be more assertive. I was never always assertive. . . . Another thing I would like to tell parents is not to be afraid to be assertive in advocating for their child, too. I think that would be important. Because if they don't do that right away, they don't feel empowered to do what they think needs to be done for their child. They will think that someone else will determine what's right, and they need to have that empowerment. So I guess another recommendation is to be assertive when you're advocating for them. (Survey 242)

Several parents couched their advice concerning advocacy within the context of being knowledgeable about their options and the legislation that supports services for children with disabilities:

My husband's much more determined that we will get what we're asking from the school system or from whoever is in charge, whoever is in charge of paying for it, I guess. And we were told she would never ever be allowed to go to a school in [another state] because [our] state would not pay for the child to go to school in [another state]. And we got her there. . . . But you know, more is possible, and the more you find out, the more people you talk to, children do get that help. . . . You go to the people who should know, and they don't know. And you have to just say, "Well, find out!" Because they don't even try to find out, which I think is the most shocking thing about the whole process for us—is that people who are supposed to be professionals . . . I thought they would be advising us, and instead you have to do all the homework and tell them what's appropriate . . . 'cuz otherwise they don't even know that it's different from any other problem or handicap or whatever. (Survey 30)

I think parents need to look more into it, that is, the laws and so forth, because we were getting a little bit of the runaround. And, like I said, we were buttin' our head against a wall with me 'cuz they more or less done what they wanted to do. And we just didn't have the knowledge then, you know, to try and fight for his needs. And I would tell the parent to look more in depth in the situation instead of just letting it go. And if there is a good school, then I would look more into a program like that than some of these programs that are through your local school. I'm not saying every local program's like that, but ours has been, and they have been to me very unhelpful in this situation. But I would seek more advice when it comes, if they got into a situation like we did. (Survey 231)

Talk to your school district, and see what they're going to provide. And fight for your kid if you need to. Go the legal route if you need to. (Survey 61)

Although advocating for a child can sometimes create an adversarial relationship between parents and professionals, there are benefits in communicating and cooperating with school personnel as part of an educational team. Recommendations included communicating with school personnel about their concerns and working with them to make sure the child is learning what he or she needs:

If I have a problem, usually I get in touch with her aide and with her speech therapist. And they work on it at school. So that there's kind of a backup when she's not there and we're having a problem, they're trying to deal with it at school. Between the three of us, we try and get it worked out. But that's really all I can say as far as advice. (Survey 211)

As far as professionals go, go to the IEP meetings. You have to. The parents need to state what they feel is going to be best for their child. They need to rely on information both from professionals and other parents. You know, don't listen to just one source. Everybody has good information. I feel that gathering information is better than just one person's point of view as to what's best for that child. (Survey 288)

Trust your instincts. Keep fighting for what you need when it comes to the school district. Approach them as your friend and not the enemy. I can't believe some of the horror stories that we hear about schools. It's unbelievable. (Survey 61)

One parent presented a good rationale for acting as an advocate for her child and reasons for overcoming the challenges that sometimes block optimal service provision:

I'd say that people should really fight for their kids, not give up, not feel like OK, well, it's too far to go over there, or that can't ever happen. . . . Just keep on advocating for what you really want for your kids because oftentimes it can happen. You just can't give up 'cuz it's really worth it. 'Cuz you see them doing so well. (Survey 80)

This mother believed that investment in her daughter now would result in a healthier, better adjusted, and more independent adult. Her comment leads to the last theme in this chapter: the importance of developing the child's positive self-concept or self-esteem.

Foster Self-Esteem

Many of the parents' comments cited earlier related to the need to love one's child, have patience, and keep the lines of communication open. These are parenting strategies that relate to the development of good self-esteem in all children. Research indicates that deaf children and adolescents who experienced social and language deprivation also exhibit deficits in self-esteem (Greenberg & Kusché, 1993). Parents addressed the importance of developing a positive self-concept for their child, especially when they could already see damage to their child's self-esteem:

> *At my school, I think there is one other student who is more profoundly deaf. I mean, I can't remember what the percentage is there, but he really feels different. And anything you can do to make [the school personnel] realize that it's important to work on the self-esteem. I think that would help a lot of things later.* (Survey 186)

One mother set her concerns about her child's self-esteem within the context of resolving her own feelings of grief. To see the mother upset about her child's hearing loss would contribute to the daughter's negative feelings about herself. She advised the following:

> *I guess I would just say, don't treat 'em any differently than you would a hearing child. Don't make the point that they can't hear—don't make it a big issue. Treat 'em like you would anything else. Do what you have to do to make sure that your child has a successful life and that they're getting the best care in school and things that they need, but don't treat 'em differently because they become, then they have a problem with their esteem, knowing that they can't hear. If their parents treat them differently, what are they gonna think about a stranger that treats them differently? Just treat 'em normal.* (Survey 211)

Several parents described situations they arranged to enhance their child's positive self-feelings. One family used sporting activities for this purpose:

> *These children can do anything they want, they just need family support. . . . She rides horses, and that really helps her, helps build her self-esteem, and they make her talk up there, you know, when she's on the*

horse, for it to walk and whoa. . . . Keep 'em involved. I mean just because they can't hear doesn't mean they can't participate in community activities. (Survey 242)

Calderon and Greenberg (1999) suggest that problems with self-esteem may be more apparent in deaf adolescents who have experienced years of social and language deficits. Parents of younger deaf children may need support to communicate effectively and encourage the development of positive self-esteem in their children. Parents of older deaf children may need guidance in facilitating peer interactions and social support for their child who may be struggling with self-identity issues.

Conclusions

When faced with the complexity and challenge represented by raising a child who is deaf or hard of hearing, many parents recognized the invaluable support they could receive from other parents. Hearing parents, especially, relied on other parents, as well as professionals, to overcome their initial feelings of shock and grief. Both hearing and deaf parents looked to other parents, hoping to gain from their experiences. This chapter provides one resource for parents to obtain advice from other parents who have "been there." The themes that emerged as central for other parents include focusing on the child first, acknowledging feelings and moving on, seeking support from other parents, becoming knowledgeable about options and resources, advocating for an appropriate education, and fostering the child's self-esteem.

Appendix D lists many resources for parents. These include parent support groups, parenting networks, and parent training centers that are supported with federal funds. The listed resources include publications, organizations, and Internet sites covering a wide range of topics and perspectives. These and other resources can provide the basis for becoming fully informed on options for deaf and hard of hearing children, as well as for making contact with people who can provide information and support.

Chapter 9
Parent to Professional: Respect Our Views

One thing that I love to hear from a professional is " . . . How can I help you?" I mean, when they look at me square in the eye, "Well, how is it that I can help you?" . . . that increases my respect for them. . . . I just appreciate them getting my input that way. (Survey 218)

Parents discover their children's hearing loss in different ways. Some suspect a hearing loss at an early age, whereas others assume their baby is hearing until someone refers them after newborn hearing screening; still others assume their baby is hearing for months or even years. Regardless of how or when they suspect the hearing loss, parents are likely to interact with pediatricians; ear, nose, and throat specialists; audiologists; deaf education specialists; occupational and physical therapists; and speech and language pathologists during the hearing evaluation and initiation of early education services. Parents depend upon these professionals to provide information, resources, support, and encouragement. Many professionals that parents encounter have little experience with young children and families. Although they have expertise in their disciplines, professionals may lack training in and experience with hearing loss in young children or with family-centered practices (Roush, Harrison, & Palsha, 1991; Roush, Harrison, Palsha, & Davidson, 1992; Stredler-Brown & Arehardt, 2000). Parents participating in the NPP reported that some professionals do not understand the major issues of deaf education and are not as helpful as they might be.

Newborn hearing screening has effected an increase in the number of infants with hearing loss and their families who enter early intervention systems. Although a family-centered service model is endorsed by federal legislation (Part C of the Individuals with Disabilities Act [IDEA]) and recommended by professional organizations (Sandall, McLean, & Smith,

158

2000), providing services that put families "in the driver's seat" is a challenge for many practitioners (Harrison, Darnhardt, & Roush, 1996). Family-centered professionals are expected to develop positive, collaborative relationships with families and consider parents as partners (Bodner-Johnson & Sass-Lehrer, 1999). Professionals should advocate for services that are consistent with family priorities and concerns and ensure that parents are the chief decision makers for their children and families.

Parents' experiences and advice are a valuable source of information for improving services. This chapter summarizes the NPP survey and interview data dealing with parents' advice to professionals. We present parents' evaluations of the support they received from professionals and others along with suggestions for how these specialists can improve the manner in which they break the news, provide information about deafness and available services, interact with parents, encourage parental involvement, and discuss communication and technology.

Parent Survey and Interview Data

In the NPP survey we asked parents about the responsiveness of program staff to their family's concerns, ideas, and questions. We also asked to what extent their services were based on their child's individual needs, whether they were active team members, and whether they felt that professionals accepted the limits on time their family could devote to the program. Responses to the survey indicate that parents were generally satisfied with the quality of the services provided (see chapter 1 and Appendix C).

Overall, parents gave high marks for the quality of the services they received. Three out of four parents reported that staff members were "always" responsive to their family's concerns. Almost 70% believed that the services they received were based on the child's individual needs. Two out of three parents said that they were active members of the team, not just listeners, and two out of three believed that the staff accepted their limits in participating in an early intervention program.

Evaluations by deaf parents and by those from minority groups, however, reveal a different picture. Compared to hearing parents, fewer deaf parents gave these services high marks. Compared to others, parents who were non-White or Hispanic were also less positive about the quality of their services. For these families, the older their child was when the hearing loss was confirmed, the less positive they were about their services.

The survey also addressed sources of support for parents. Teachers were rated highest as sources of support, followed by spouses, therapists, other parents, and deaf adults. Doctors were less helpful to parents than others. Parents with children who had additional conditions, minority parents, and parents with less education reported less overall support than their comparison groups. Interviews provided more in-depth understanding of parents' perspectives about services and elicited many suggestions for professionals on how to improve the assistance they provide to families, encourage more active involvement by families, and generally improve services.

Breaking the News

Most parents vividly recall the events surrounding the discovery of a child's hearing loss. They can recount in detail who broke the news and how they did so. Many parents were critical of pediatricians who disregarded their concerns and did not quickly refer them to specialists for a hearing test. The most frequent piece of advice these parents gave was "listen to parents":

I think pediatricians should listen to what the parents are saying and make a referral or whatever, regardless, just to rule it out. I think that needs to be standardized. You know, when people come in and say "I have a little concern," it needs to be standard that they make that referral. They oftentimes are just looking at the child and saying, "Oh, he's fine." They will clap their hands or pop their fingers. (Focus Group 3)

First and foremost, they must remember . . . these people are scared. These people don't know what's going on—don't know what to expect. Talk to them like ordinary people—no matter what their income, religion, background, anything. Just sit down face to face and, you know, let them . . . know everything. Quit just, you know, putting people off. That is very important. (Survey 16)

Some parents were upset that their doctors were not well informed about hearing loss. The medical doctor I saw—I'm still angry. Urge them to become better informed, not rely on us to inform them. (Focus Group 1)

Usually you have to find things out for yourself—and usually after there's been a big mistake. (Focus Group 1)

Parents whose children were hard of hearing rather than deaf most often expressed the concern that their doctor missed their child's hearing loss:

The pediatrician who [my son] first was going to . . . he was very unprofessional, because I was expressing my concerns, and he just kept telling me that I was a worried and paranoid parent, which turned out not to be so. (Survey 185)

Parents stressed that they know their children better than the professionals:

You know, a parent usually knows their kids more or better than the doctor who doesn't see them all the time. You know, if they have a real concern, you know, listen to them . . . not tell them it's all in their head. . . . That presents frustration right there . . . because you're trying to explain to somebody that, you know, you're noticing something that's not right, but no—and they're supposed to be professional enough to listen to you and try to help you. (Survey 251)

How the message is communicated is also very important:

I would say that you have to listen to what that parent is saying. . . . If you are going to be the bearer of bad news, it is important how you deliver that information. . . . I think that they're that initial person to make that link

for you. They can make or break that experience. . . . It's going to be a
shock no matter what, but to just give people hope. (Focus Group 3)

I think it's very important to sit people down to share that information.
. . . I think they need to . . . be able to slot time and not think so much
about that next client that's getting ready to come in . . . instead of just a
15-minute consultation. . . . I had a lot of questions, and I felt like giving
me that information over the phone was inappropriate. (Focus Group 3)

And another thing, I guess, for professionals is not only to listen but to give
them adequate time. That is very important to me. If I feel that they are
rushed, I won't try to take their time. So, I guess, when you're meeting
with parents, give enough time, and sometimes it takes a little more time
for them to unwind or feel comfortable with a stranger. So if . . . I feel
they are listening intently to me and they have enough time, I'll open up
and I'll say things. And . . . it will help me to trust them if they do care
about me and my child. (Survey 242)

The Next Step

By the time the hearing loss is identified, many parents have experienced
a roller-coaster ride of emotions. Whether newborn hearing screening
suggests a hearing loss or the parents feel—after months of suspicion—that
something is not quite right with their baby, parents need both support
and information to take the next steps after the hearing loss is finally confirmed. Advice from families in the NPP is similar to that expressed by
parents in a study by Luterman and Kurtzer-White (1999) assessing parents' opinions about early detection of hearing loss and appropriate
follow-up. In that study parents identified a need for contact with other
parents, unbiased information, time to process information, and skillful and
supportive professionals.

For many parents this is an emotional experience, and they appreciate
working with professionals who are sensitive to their feelings. One parent
suggested that counselors be involved with parents when their child's
hearing loss is confirmed:

I would have loved to [sit] with someone like a counselor or something at that time instead of the audiologist. The audiologist said, "Well, you know, he has a severe-to-profound hearing loss and duh, duh, duh, duh" . . . and just gave us the facts and said, "Now he's gotta go to [city] and have a brain stem test, and we'll set that up as fast as possible." I would rather have had some counselor sit down and say, "Well, these are the services that are available, and you have a choice. We have . . . this school does this and this school does that, and he's still young and . . . we have services where someone can come to your house and someone can do this . . . and all these things are available to you. And we'd be glad to answer all of your questions" . . . and just kind of ease us into it. We were told and kind of left on our own. (Survey 65)

Well, they definitely have to be sensitive to the parents who are emotional, like myself. I bawled like a baby for the first week. I was calling them constantly, and they were reassuring me. They have to be sensitive because it's a traumatic thing for the parent. I was, like, traumatized because I didn't know what I was headed for in the future. (Survey 76)

Parents want professionals to be sensitive to their feelings and understand they may need time to adjust to new information:

When you walk out with your head in your lap because you are very depressed . . . to say, "It's not the end of the world, and if you need to call me again, you can. I would be happy to talk with you" and "Why don't you next week sometime when you are feeling like it to give this place a call?" You know, that helps. (Focus Group 3)

Another parent advised the following:

Give the parents time to deal with their child being deaf in the first place 'cuz . . . you know, we still get brokenhearted about it and . . . it's something . . . that's taken us time to come to grips with. (Survey 231)

Advice from parents was that professionals should just ask them what they need:

Just start with asking them what would be most helpful. Asking the parents because it's hard to know or to assume that every parent wants to do everything possible. . . . The thing I would say is just ask them. And you may have to ask them every other month because this month I might want to do everything possible and next month I just might not be able to. (Survey 73)

Provide Information about Deafness and Available Services

Parents stressed the importance of being well informed and encouraged professionals to share as much information as possible with them. Some parents suggested every doctor's office have a pamphlet with basic information about hearing loss and what to do. Other suggestions included a resource phone number to call, lists of names and numbers of schools, information centers, and contact information for other parents with deaf or hard of hearing children in their community. Many parents want resources for financial assistance. They wanted someone to share information with them in person and thought it was important for professionals to give them the name of someone to contact after leaving the office:

Telling parents where they can get information—whether it's periodicals or inservice or with other parents and perhaps . . . if there are those that don't have the time or the interest to keep up through periodicals or inservice, putting them in touch with parents, other parents can empower them. And I guess I would recommend that, because just knowing you're not alone . . . sharing stories helps [parents] to be more assertive in what they feel is right for their child. Otherwise they don't know and if some other parent feels the same way, they'll go, "Yeah, I wasn't so far off." Putting them in touch with other parents and an information center or periodicals or inservice. (Survey 242)

Parents recommended that professionals put aside their own agenda when dealing with families:

So when this lady came to me, and she heard my concerns, she gave me information on what my concerns were. She did not come in with a packet of . . . "Why don't you read this and this?" She made it specific to me. And that's where I believe instead of coming in with . . . "Oh boy, they need more information," let it come from the parents first. Let them identify the problem, and then give them the information. (Survey 242)

How to Interact with Parents

A central goal of a family-centered approach is to promote family strengths and enhance the family's sense of well-being. Boyd and Dunst (1993) identify professional behaviors that support families' feelings of self-efficacy and control. Among the behaviors they identify are effective listening skills, effective communication, respect, and honesty. Families that the NPP interviewed repeated many of these ideas.

Several parents commented on the ways in which professionals (both medical and educational) interact with parents and ways they might be more effective:

I guess we worked with such wonderful people that I never really had to think about it. I would just say . . . keep the lines of communication open and explain—say, for an evaluation-type process, exactly what has to be done and why a particular test is important. Just keep the lines of communication open and . . . just be available . . . answer questions. Don't talk down to people, but . . . also explain things in terms that people can understand. Be positive, but not overly optimistic, you know, be realistic, in other words. Just develop a good relationship. (Survey 224)

Also commenting on the importance of effective communication, another parent added:

I think the main thing would be keeping the line[s] of communication open and listening to what the parent has to say and paying attention to it. I've been pretty lucky that most of the professionals that I've dealt with have been . . . pretty wonderful. (Survey 257)

Again emphasizing the importance of listening to parents, another interviewee remarked:

I liked it when they sat down with me and listened. . . . So much happened in a short amount of time, and I needed to bring [my son] here and there for testing. But what was so nice is when they would interview me or they listened so intently. I had a lot of concerns and a lot of concerns with placement, and the hearing impaired teacher again listened. And she absorbed what I was saying and . . . and so I believe [what] they can do is to stop and listen to parents. (Survey 242)

Be willing to listen to them [parents] and what their concerns are. And to try to help the parent become better informed and becoming more involved instead of just assuming that parents can't understand what the problem is and making a diagnosis and saying this is what you need to do without explaining things. I've been through that many times. Where you'll have somebody say, "OK, this is what you need to do," and walk out of the room. And I'm saying, "Well, why?" They get really offended if you question. Say, maybe I don't agree or maybe we should try something else. (Survey 75)

Respect was a recurring theme in the comments of the parents we interviewed:

I guess the main thing that I think a lot of professionals forget when they're working with families is . . . not that I think they should treat them as though they're family . . . but I think not treat 'em as though they're just another face. You know, really listen to what the parents are saying. I mean . . . the teachers go to school to . . . have college training and things to teach a child, but a parent really knows their child. And I think they know better what works for their child than the teacher does from reading it in a book. . . . So I guess the most is just to try and make the family and child feel like they're important and not just another face or another file in their desk. (Survey 211)

I didn't like being petted on the head and given sort of pat, rote answers to problems and issues that I was dealing with. . . . You get the impression that social workers and people in the business sort of refer to parents as in the third person as though I was sort of childlike, like my child was. And if I had just been given credit for being a reasonably intelligent person who was interested in being involved and aggressive in helping my child, I would've appreciated that. (Survey 121)

Parents felt that some professionals act as if they have power and control:

The specialists just see themselves as the authority, not only over the child and the condition, but over the parent. (Survey 75)

One observer believes that parents of deaf children often feel powerless and experience a "sense of lack of control" that can lead to a whole series of negative consequences for children (Schlesinger, 1992, p. 39). The following mother described how her feelings of powerlessness began very early and how professionals might return some control to parents:

When [your] child is first diagnosed, you feel like all the control has been ripped out of your hands. Everything is now in someone else's hands, and the most important thing seems to be to give some element of control or choice, maybe that "choice" is a better word, some element of choice back to the parent and also to the children, so the parents feel like no one's treating them like a child. (Survey 348)

Another parent suggested that professionals would be more effective if they would just "get down on the parents' level":

I mean, I know they're professionals, but they still need to kinda get on the parents' level, you know, and what that parent is feeling and what they're trying to deal with . . . which you can still do that and maintain that professional thing. (Parent comment, American Society for Deaf Children Conference, July 2000)

Parents felt strongly about the importance of honesty in the parent-professional relationship. Even if the news was not good, parents wanted professionals to tell them everything and give it to them straight:

I guess to just listen to parents . . . and, I guess, tell them everything. . . . Everything is not always gonna be a good answer or what we want to hear, but the truth is always the best thing. (Survey 185)

I also would have appreciated . . . as many facts as were available. Because a lot of times when you have a child who is very ill or has an uncertain future, the medical profession is hesitant to just tell you what they're thinking. And so you end up worrying about things you don't even have to worry about. (Survey 121)

One parent complained that professionals led her to believe that her child would learn to talk if he wore his hearing aids daily:

And they were saying, well, if he wears these, he's gonna be picking up speech left and right. And, well, with his type of hearing loss at that time, we didn't know that was impossible. So we were thinking, well, if he puts these on, his speech is gonna be—he's just gonna be picking up words left and right, and we found out that wasn't the case. And I think . . . we really got aggravated because they got our hopes up about that. Be more

honest about it. And let the parents know that they may or they may not.
. . . And . . . they kinda led us to believe that . . . he wears these, no
problem, he's gonna be able to talk normal just like everybody else . . .
and we found out that wasn't the case. And that was pretty disturbing.
(Survey 231)

Many parents were very satisfied with the interactions they had with teachers. Their sentiments might be summed up by this parent's comments:

Well . . . I have no complaints. They were just wonderful. I couldn't give
them any advice. They . . . were open, I mean they made me feel wel-
come in the school; they were willing to talk anytime—all the time with
me. (Survey 202)

Encouraging Parental Involvement

Parental involvement is widely regarded as a safeguard against delays in communication or in cognitive or socioemotional development that may otherwise materialize with a child with a hearing loss. Several researchers (e.g., Bodner-Johnson, 1986; Calderon, Bargones, & Sidman, 1998; Moeller, 2000) have documented the power of parental involvement and suggest that parents who are actively involved in their child's early development can moderate the potentially harmful effects of late identification and a delay in intervention.

We asked parents how professionals can encourage more involvement. They mentioned the importance of cooperation and feeling like equal members of the team that develops the Individualized Family Service Plan (IFSP) or the Individualized Educational Plan (IEP):

When the goals are written . . . I think they should be consulting with the
parents right along . . . to write a reasonable goal. . . . They are with
your children 6 hours out of the day; they know what your child is capa-
ble of as well as yourself. So this should be a team effort. (Survey 13)

Families often receive services from different agencies and school programs. Cooperation among professionals makes it easier for parents to participate effectively with the team:

> The people in [the school district] know they can call the people in [the
> city where the school for deaf children is located] if they have a question
> or if a problem develops like that. So I guess another bit of advice would
> be to work like a team. Nobody's any greater or any smarter or any less
> smart or something than anybody else. . . . We're all in there [together],
> and the goal is to do what's best for the child. And I guess we're just lucky
> that everybody's got that in mind. (Survey 224)

> It was so nice to know that everybody . . . really does have his best inter-
> est in mind, and we're all going through the same challenges with him
> when it comes to behavior. And so it's just nice to really work on a true
> IEP team. Sometimes you go to the IEP meetings and feel like you're just
> there. They really don't have any of your input. And I had heard a rumor
> through the grapevine that one school district we were in—that they had
> everything in the IEP planned out before the parents ever showed up.
> And I felt like that when I went to IEP meetings at that school district. I
> was never part of a team. (Survey 257).

> We always felt like we could come into the classroom at any point. We
> could participate; we could be part of—they weren't just working with
> the child—they were working with the whole family. So there was a lot
> of ongoing communication, like I said, we would talk daily or every other
> day . . . about this or that and how's it going and what do you need, and
> how's she doing and this sort of thing . . . and how are the siblings doing
> and how's your husband doing? You know, all that kind of stuff. So it was
> almost like a family school in a sense because . . . they worked with all of
> us, with all of our different needs. And so I think that was tremendously
> helpful. (Survey 80)

Because parents sometimes live far from the programs where they
receive services, their participation may be difficult. Regular communica-

tion and the scheduling of events at times that are convenient for parents were recommendations we heard from one mother:

Well, at this time, we're communicating through the communication book we send back and forth. If there's any problem, why, we pick up the phone. And it's pretty hard for me and his father, both working and the distance. . . . I know that's hard to do 'cuz they [the professionals] have family, too—and more weekend events. . . . At the . . . times they have a lot of these events on are just impossible for the parents to be there. . . . Maybe having picnics once in a while on a Saturday . . . maybe getting together somewhere having a picnic where everybody can get together and, you know, be more involved. . . . But . . . like I said, it's really hard through the week for people working, and the distance of where they live, too, makes a difference. But as long as we can keep that communication by phone and by notebook . . . that helps a lot. (Survey 231)

Whereas some parents think their school programs welcome parents, others feel differently:

I feel like they [the school for deaf children] don't have enough parent involvement. Sometimes I feel like when I go to visit her at school, some- times I feel like I'm intruding. . . . I mean, I like that they're very protec- tive . . . and I'm not saying that they should let anybody in at any time, but they do have strict policies on if you become a volunteer, even parents . . . have to have references to fill out these forms [laughter]. And that's wonderful because it's for my child's protection, also, but . . . there have been a couple of situations where I wanted to go on field trips or I want- ed just to drop by . . . her classes, and I wasn't allowed to go on the field trip. . . . They would use this excuse or that. (Survey 317)

Don't try to intimidate us when we come around. 'Cause there are some teachers who hate for the parents to come around and be involved. They want to do their thing in private. . . . I think they probably feel like we're hovering over and watching, but that's our child. And I want to make sure

things are done right. Don't make me feel intimidated 'cause, for me, it
won't work. Some people it will intimidate, but it don't work with me.
(Survey 334)

Opportunities for parents to get together make some parents feel more involved:

Support groups, monthly, biweekly meetings where parents can sit around
and discuss their situations and what they would like to see incorporated
in the curriculum. That helps a lot—plus it makes, I believe, the parents
closer and the children closer. The parents . . . the group that we've got
over there is just tremendous—parents that we've had . . . it's just been
great to get together and talk about different problems they've had with
their children, how they've handled it. (Survey 24)

Other parents felt strongly that professionals cannot force parental involvement and that the interest must come from the parents themselves. On the other hand, some parents felt that professionals need to be sure that parents understand the importance of being involved:

I guess I would tell professionals to . . . drill it into a parent's head that the
child's prognosis—their accomplishments—can only be determined by the
involvement of the parents. . . . I feel that professionals could do a better
job at that. They kinda, "Oh yeah, you know, it's sad," they kinda tiptoe
around it instead of saying, "OK, this is what you got dealt. . . . Do
somethin.'" So, however, they could do that diplomatically [laughter] and
get their point across. (Survey 293)

Discussing Communication and Technology

Families must often make decisions about the communication approach they wish to use with their child before they have a chance to understand their child's communicative abilities and the options (see chapter 2). Parents have many questions and find that some professionals have biases or do not provide all of the information they need for informed decisions.

Some parents expressed concerns about their ability to learn sign language. Pressure to acquire signing skills quickly and to be able to communicate effectively may be difficult and frustrating for some families (Lynas, 1999). According to the parents we interviewed, sign language classes do not always address the needs of parents, and parents urged the professionals to be patient as they learned to sign:

As far as the teacher, I think a lot of it is communication and . . . they've got to understand the parents' frustration, too, of this . . . and just like we were talking about the sign language . . . like I said, up until we found out Alex was deaf, we weren't familiar with being around deaf people. And as far as learning the language, I mean it's hard to me, and it can be frustrating. . . . I sometimes . . . feel there are a few people who expect you to learn it overnight and really think if you aren't fluent with it. . . . I really think that some of them try to push you too hard for that and . . . we've got to give it time and let the parents . . . feel comfortable with it. (Survey 231)

Parents also appreciated a patient approach in teaching them how to manage hearing aids and other hearing technologies:

So they were really good about the way they explained . . . everything and helped us as far as his hearing aids themselves, because . . . we had no idea how they worked or . . . what we had to do to care for them and how to put them in even and that kinda thing. (Survey 21)

Parents commented on the importance of flexibility on the part of the professionals and the program so that if one approach or technology is not working professionals will accommodate to the child's communication needs:

> *Derick's hearing equipment did not work right, so he went almost a week*
> *without sound until we could find out what the problem was. He was*
> *strictly in that oral class. . . . I went to the school that day, and I was*
> *almost in tears because Derick was sitting there like this—because he*
> *couldn't understand. . . . I was told that we couldn't switch him. [They]*
> *couldn't accommodate. I had a hard time with that. He was in a situa-*
> *tion where he didn't have somebody to sign to him or give him that one*
> *on one. . . . Hearing aids and cochlear implants or whatever devices you*
> *are using could malfunction. If that child was depending on sound, and*
> *they're not able to grasp or whatever, I think this program doesn't have as*
> *much flexibility with that.* (Focus Group 3)

One parent described a very helpful seminar on communication approaches. Another parent praised professionals who recommended various videos and books on communication methodologies. Deciding on a communication approach takes time and is most effective when it is a collaborative process between families and professionals (Moeller & Condon, 1994).

General Recommendations

Implementing a family-centered philosophy requires that professionals support a general perspective rather than applying a prescribed set of strategies (Bailey, 1996). Families differ, and the context for services varies. Thus an approach that is successful with one family may not be successful with another. No single prescribed set of behaviors defines a family-centered philosophy (McWilliam, Winton, & Crais, 1996). Interviews with parents reflect the complexity of providing services with the right amount of direction and encouragement. Four general recommendations emerged from the interviews that demonstrate the complexities of the challenges facing professionals:

- Be direct—but don't tell us what to do
- Tell the truth and be honest—but also be hopeful and encouraging
- Be knowledgeable—but admit when you don't know the answer
- Don't overwhelm—but don't hold back information

Be Direct—But Don't Tell Us What to Do

I don't know that they could've been more sensitive, but they could've been more direct with me because, I don't know if this is true for all parents, but in that first couple of years when you're hit with all of this medical stuff and running to the doctors and . . . getting them tested and equipment . . . I could've used direction. I wasn't getting it from the doctors. . . . Teachers and all like that [should] be always up-front and tell the parents what's goin' on at all times . . . and always tell them . . . "We suggest that this needs to be done or that needs to be done." Don't leave 'em in the dark. . . . Just tell 'em . . . "This is what's gotta be done." (Survey 73)

Other parents suggest that professionals may go too far in telling parents what to do:

Well, the first thing is just to become as well informed as you can about . . . the type of hearing loss, about the different methods. I mean instead of being told—I meant that's the thing I've heard a lot of parents [say] that audiologists or somebody just say . . . "Here's how—what you should do." I think there needs to be made available to them what the options available to them are . . . and let them read the reports to educate themselves and let them make the decision. (Survey 75)

Tell the Truth—But Also Be Hopeful and Encouraging

They're wise if they don't try to tell you. That was one of the greatest things is they told me right up front: "We don't know [what will happen]." Instead of trying to tell me, well, something dreadful, they just said, "Well, you know, we just don't know." You can live with that a little bit better than you can [with] . . . "Gee, your son is never gonna walk." The best thing that the educators can do is just to be honest with parents. Gosh, you know, I really respect people who are just honest with me. I can, even when they fail, if they're honest with me, I can accept that. So . . . that'll go a long way, if they're straightforward. (Survey 73)

It was their whole approach—it was very positive. They were always focused on the things she could do and the things she did well. It was just . . . you're spending all of this time with specialists, and they're telling you all of the things that she can't do, won't be able to do. (Survey 75)

Be Knowledgeable—But Admit When You Don't Know the Answer

If every story of every parent I have met whose child is deaf wasn't the same, I would say it's just us, but every parent said their pediatrician had not a clue or brushed you off. (Focus Group 3)

I just really wish that the doctors . . . were more familiar . . . even the otolaryngologists in our area were the very people who looked me in the face and said, "It is not a hearing problem." (Survey, 344)

Don't Overwhelm—But Don't Hold Back Information

I felt like at times I needed more, and other times I felt overwhelmed. So, well, it's nobody's fault. It's just different things change, and your abilities vary, so you want to give parents everything they need, but you don't want to throw too much at them. And so I guess you just have to ask, "OK, look, what do you need right now? This is what we see your child needs right now, but what do you want to do?" (Survey 73)

Finding the "golden mean" is difficult in any effort involving human relations, and this is no exception. The appropriate approach for one parent may antagonize another. "Being direct" in one situation may seem "insensitive" in another. Experience, trial and error, and open-mindedness all help. Above all, approaching every family with the knowledge that they are different from every other family, getting to know each individual, and developing positive relationships are fundamental to effective parent-professional relationships.

Professionals need to know how to provide effective family-centered services to all families with deaf and hard of hearing children. From the first professional who breaks the news to the team of professionals working with the family to help strengthen their resources and to select and implement services, the effectiveness of the parent-professional relationship hinges on knowledge, sensitivity, and interaction skills. Parents expect professionals to be unbiased and honest and to possess exceptional communication skills. They value professionals who listen to their concerns, solicit their opinions, and respect and support their decisions. Professionals must be mindful of individual circumstances, expectations, and responses and examine their interaction styles to determine how best to support parents' quest for better lives for the child and the family.

Chapter 10
Concluding Thoughts

Just as we have seen dramatic changes in education and technology for deaf and hard of hearing children in the past 30 years, we will likely see far-reaching changes in the coming decades. It seems certain that newborn hearing screening will indeed become universal. Already 70% of all newborns are being screened for hearing loss at birth (National Center for Hearing Assessment and Management, 2002). Perhaps the children deriving the most benefit from this change are those with a minimal hearing loss that in the past might well have gone undetected for many months. Increased use of cochlear implants is one of the most dramatic changes in the recent past, and educators can expect to see many more implanted children in the future. Improvements in computers, TTYs, video communication, real-time voice-to-print devices, and related technologies will pose new issues and opportunities for children and their families (Meadow-Orlans, 2002b).

Current trends are likely to continue, perhaps with accelerating effects on the demographics of families with deaf and hard of hearing children. By 2050 the Hispanic population is expected to triple and the African American population to increase by 70%. More mothers of young children will be working outside the home, and more children will be growing up in single-parent homes if present trends continue. Educators must be prepared to serve more children from such families.

Highlights of the NPP Survey

Every parent and child characteristic that the NPP survey examined exhibits great variation. Although averages are reported, these do not give a complete picture. The 404 children the survey represents were born in 1989 and 1990, before the adoption of newborn hearing screening legislation. Nevertheless, the average age at which the deaf children's hearing loss was identified—14.5 months—is considerably below that of 10 years earlier. Identified at an average age of 28.6 months, hard of hearing children experienced unacceptable delays.

About one third of survey children have conditions in addition to deafness—a proportion similar to that reported in Gallaudet's annual survey for many years. However, the proportion of children identified by their parents as having behavioral problems—about 9%—is higher than the annual survey figures for this age group, suggesting that parents may be more willing than teachers to label young children.

Although 60% of parents reported they were given a choice in their child's early intervention program, 40% had no choice. In about 25% of programs, speech alone was the communication approach; sign language plus speech was used in two thirds. The remainder was divided among sign language alone, Cued Speech, and speech plus cues.

Overall, parents evaluated program services very positively. However, significant differences were found for some subgroups, with hearing parents more positive than deaf or hard of hearing parents, and White parents more positive than Hispanic, non-White, or mixed-race parents. Two thirds of parents believed their child's teachers had been "very helpful." Spouses were identified as the next most helpful source of support, with medical personnel near the bottom of a considerable list. Minority families and those without a college education reported lower levels of support than White families and those with some college education.

Communication Decisions

Communication issues are of the utmost concern to parents: "How will we communicate with our child?" "Will she ever learn to talk?" "How will he be able to communicate with others?" Communication methods are among the first decisions parents face, and they quickly discover that professionals and other parents can have strong and sometimes conflicting opinions. Their choices are determined by their beliefs, expectations for their children, and their knowledge of deaf people. The need to speak with hearing people in the "hearing world" led many parents to choose speech as their primary communication method. Others based their decisions on their understanding of the benefits and limitations of different communication approaches. Parents also considered how well their children could hear and their progress in learning to speak. It was not always easy for parents to get clear and comprehensive information about communication methods. Some parents found books, other parents, and deaf adults more helpful than professionals. They wanted their children to be able to communicate with both hearing and deaf people and to be able to choose, as adults, the method that would be best for them.

Most children used both speech and signs at home. Deaf children were more likely than hard of hearing children to use some sign language. Few children used Cued Speech or an auditory verbal approach. Many parents had difficulty finding appropriate sign language classes and becoming fluent signers. The desire to communicate with their children led many to use every available mode: signs, speech, fingerspelling, cues, gestures, and body language. They were more concerned with the message than with the mode.

Hard of Hearing Children

The major reasons mothers gave for the delayed diagnosis of their child's hearing loss were their failure to suspect it because of the child's speechreading skills, the child's intermittent responses to sound, and physicians' reluctance to make referrals for assessment. These parents had the same reactions to identification of hearing loss as the hearing parents of deaf children: grief, self-blame, denial, and acceptance, with a focus on the child's positive assets and attributes. Several parents detailed their concerns for a child's behavioral problems or low self-image. Some attributed these difficulties to the long delay in identifying hearing loss. Despite problems in obtaining services, most parents spoke positively about their children: "She really lets people into her heart," "She's the light of my life," "He's really a delightful boy."

Additional Conditions

The provision of services to children with a hearing loss and conditions such as developmental delay, visual impairment, cerebral palsy, or behavioral problems presents special challenges for professionals and the families they serve. Parents recounted multiple visits to doctors and hospitals, fears that their child might not "make it," and gratitude for small developmental achievements. Sometimes an additional condition led to early identification, but sometimes it masked the hearing loss and thus delayed identification. The range of age at identification for these children was greater than for others.

Parents had to acquire a wide range of information (e.g., about how to get and deal with professional help for conditions such as cerebral palsy or temper tantrums). Services that were provided in the home or that directly addressed multiple needs were especially valuable. In some cases services related to hearing loss were not provided because of a child's behavioral problems. A therapist who could sign helped one family whose adopted child had a history of abuse. Teams of professionals with knowledge of deafness and sign language can be helpful for families and their children with multiple conditions.

Deaf Parents

The experiences and opinions of deaf and hearing parents differed markedly, starting with the identification of the child's hearing loss. Most deaf parents recognized that their children might be deaf or hard of hearing and tested them informally at home soon after birth. Deafness was usually met with acceptance and even joy, not regret or sorrow. Deaf parents wanted their children to wear hearing aids, use speech, and learn to speechread. However, they were less insistent than hearing parents that the children wear hearing aids. Some regretted that they had too little professional assistance in encouraging a child's speech and wished for advice about discipline or other concerns. All of the deaf parents signed: Some used American Sign Language (without speech), and others used sign language with speech. Several remarked that teachers and other hearing professionals working with deaf children should improve their signing skills. They hoped that teachers would have the same expectations for deaf children as for hearing children.

Children with Cochlear Implants

Eleven percent of the children whose parents responded to the NPP survey had received cochlear implants. Two thirds of these parents reported that the implant was "very satisfactory," and another 21%, "somewhat satisfactory." All but 3 of 44 children (7%) were using the implant at the time of the survey. Parents' motivations for the surgery included a desire to give their children "every opportunity"—to develop speech, to succeed academically, and to promote social development and communication with hearing and deaf people. Some parents reported that members of the Deaf community advised them against seeking an implant. Most parents seemed satisfied with the help they had received and reported significantly more support than parents whose children did not have implants. Three quarters of the mothers and 65% of the fathers used some signs or cues with their implanted children, although they were frequently advised not to do so. The expense of implant surgery made it an option only for well-to-do families or those with good medical insurance.

Minority Families

The rapid growth of the minority population makes the task of serving its deaf and hard of hearing children an urgent one. The hearing loss of Hispanic and Asian/Pacific children was identified significantly later than that of White or Black children, in part because physicians dismissed parents' suspicions of hearing loss. The later diagnosis of Hispanic children may also result from language differences or because medical services were less accessible to Spanish speakers.

Although minority parents, like others, felt shock and grief about a child's hearing loss, religion was often helpful to them. The support of the extended family was more common for Black than for Hispanic parents, several of whom had relocated far from home to obtain services for their child.

Minority parents were generally less satisfied with their services than were White parents. They felt it necessary to advocate for their children and feared discrimination. Minority households were often supported by one poorly paid person. Low incomes, distance, and scheduling conflicts often made participation in school programs difficult. When services were provided in a culturally sensitive manner close to home, parents expressed higher levels of satisfaction.

Advice to Other Parents

Parents welcomed opportunities to interact with other parents in formal support groups, informal contacts, or Internet exchanges. The most consistent advice they offered was to "treat the child as a child first." Parents reported that it is not only important to acknowledge grief and shock but also essential to get beyond those feelings and focus on the child's best interests. Hearing parents found the support of other parents and professionals helpful. Deaf parents were less concerned about their child's hearing loss but more concerned about obtaining appropriate services, often because of their own negative childhood experiences.

Parents are responsible for learning about hearing loss and securing appropriate services for their children. Both hearing and deaf parents recommended consulting members of the Deaf community, other parents, and professionals. Appendix D lists many associations and agencies that provide resources—many of which are available on the Internet. Parents emphasized the importance of a complete, unbiased picture of options for a deaf or hard of hearing child, especially with regard to complex and controversial communication and educational choices. "The most important thing for parents to know is what is in the best interest for the child, not for themselves" (Survey 376).

Finally, parents acknowledged the necessity of playing an active role in decisions that concern their child. Professionals can do only so much: The family is the child's main source of support. Parents viewed regular visits to school programs as important. Assertive parents are more effective advocates when they understand service options and have positive relationships with professionals.

Advice to Professionals

Parents agreed that their experiences with professionals had been very favorable. Teachers were most frequently helpful during their child's early years; professionals with limited knowledge of deafness issues are less help-ful. Parents were critical of doctors who ignored their concerns and failed to recognize their child's hearing loss. Parents advised professionals to be aware of the implications of hearing loss and to give parents time to process diagnostic information. Sensitivity to cultural background, lan-guage, income, and family preferences was important. Parents stressed the need for professionals to improve their communication skills and to respect parents' concerns. They appreciated professionals who were straightforward and honest, put them in touch with other parents, and gave them useful information. They were angry with those who avoided the truth or provided inaccurate information. They wanted to be partners in their child's education as members of an educational team. As family cir-cumstances change, professionals may find it difficult to keep abreast of the family's needs. Parents respond to this by saying "Just ask us."

The Future for Deaf and Hard of Hearing Children and Their Parents

Because of expanding technological and educational options, one does not require a crystal ball to predict a brighter future for tomorrow's deaf and hard of hearing children. However, many of the issues and concerns this book raises will not disappear. An infant's hearing loss will continue to be an unhappy reality for hearing parents. Families will confront many choic-es for which they are not prepared. They will still need to make decisions about a communication mode and educational placement. Early interven-tion specialists will need to be trained and to retrain themselves to meet the challenges of different kinds of children in their programs and to help parents deal with the long-term implications of new technologies. Researchers will need to evaluate the consequences of changing tech-nologies and educational programming and to design research that is responsive to changing family demographics. Parents and professionals of the future, like those of the past, must apply all of their creative talents to ensure that deaf and hard of hearing children have the opportunity to real-ize their full potential.

Research Methodology: Design and Conduct of the National Parent Project

Methodological Approach

At each stage of the project we made an effort to include input from parents and teachers of young deaf and hard of hearing children, incorporating their views and participation (Mertens, 1998; Mertens & McLaughlin, 1995). The combination of survey, individual interviews, and focus group interviews provides a broad perspective as well as an in-depth understanding of individual family situations. The personal family experiences that the interviews and focus groups produced offer a context for the quantitative data from the survey. An advantage of qualitative data is that parents' words provide more rich detail of children and their families than the quantitative data alone can supply. From the interviews and analyses of the survey data, patterns emerged regarding both general and individual responses to the early intervention process.

The Research Team
Senior Researchers

The research team included a social scientist (Meadow-Orlans), a research and evaluation specialist (Mertens), and an early childhood teacher educator (Sass-Lehrer), who collaborated in the overall design and analysis of the study. Parents of deaf and hard of hearing children provided advice on the content as well as the format of the questionnaire for the survey phase of the project. As the data analyses proceeded and results were presented at workshops and conferences, deaf and hearing parents of deaf and hard of hearing children provided important insights into the findings from both the survey and interview portions of the project (Sass-Lehrer, Meadow-Orlans, Mertens, Scott-Olson, & Steinmetz, 1999; Sass-Lehrer,

Meadow-Orlans, Mertens, & Scott-Olson, 1999; Meadow-Orlans, Sass-Lehrer, & Mertens, 2000).

Graduate Assistants

As the project progressed, the research team expanded to include four Gallaudet University graduate students specializing in family-centered early education. Kimberley Scott-Olson entered survey data on a computer and, with Selena Steinmetz, interviewed parents, transcribed and entered interview data, and worked with the senior members of the team to establish a coding system. Jennifer Pittaway and Susan Medina assisted with library searches and with the printing and organizing of interview transcripts. Scott-Olson also coauthored chapter 7, and Pittaway helped to prepare the list of resources in Appendix D. The senior researchers benefited from the multiple perspectives and talents of the students, and the students benefited from the opportunity to participate in an ongoing research project with parents of deaf children.

Collecting the Survey Data

Program Sampling Plan

Gallaudet University's Center for Assessment and Demographic Studies (CADS) has conducted the Annual Survey of Deaf and Hard of Hearing Children and Youth for more than 30 years, maintaining a database with information on approximately 48,000 children enrolled in special education programs throughout the United States (Schildroth & Hotto, 1993). CADS provided a listing of programs enrolling children born in 1989 and 1990, together with information on the number of students in this age range and a summary of group characteristics. In the 1994–1995 school year, 3,744 children born in 1989 and 1990 were reported to the annual survey, enrolled in more than 500 different educational programs. A program sampling ensured representation of all geographic regions, program types, and program sizes, designed to yield about half of the eligible programs.

In March 1996 we mailed letters to programs serving 15 students or more, describing the purpose of the survey. A sample questionnaire and a return form indicating willingness to participate and the number of surveys required (in English and in Spanish) were also enclosed. Similar letters were sent to programs serving fewer students, enclosing multiple questionnaires, parent letters, and postage-paid envelopes. We requested that these be distributed to parents of all of the children in the targeted age group.

Participation was requested from 269 programs. One program had closed; 16 had no children ages 6 and 7 years currently enrolled. Of the remaining 252 programs, 20 were unwilling or unable to participate, and 95 did not respond to the query letter. Thus, 137 programs (54% of those contacted and eligible) agreed to distribute questionnaires to parents. We then mailed a total of 1,147 questionnaires to those programs. Although some were probably not distributed to parents, 404 (35%) were returned. This is not as high a response rate as we had hoped for, but it is not surprising considering our lack of control over the distribution of materials. In any case, respondents are similar to the children born in 1989 and 1990 who were reported to the annual survey.

Characteristics of NPP Respondents

Geographic distribution is similar to that in the CADS annual survey, with questionnaires returned from 39 states plus the District of Columbia. Somewhat underrepresented are California (8.8%; cf. 12.4%) and Texas (9.9%; cf. 14.2%). Somewhat overrepresented are Utah (5.7%; cf. 2.1%) and Maryland (5.0%; cf. 1.5%). The distribution of children by sex is similar in the two databases: Males account for 55% of CADS participants and 56% of National Parent Project (NPP) participants. Whites account for 67% of the NPP respondents and 61% of CADS annual survey respondents.

Mothers most often completed the survey forms (84%); mothers together with fathers completed an additional 5%. Fathers alone completed 6% of the questionnaires; other relatives, guardians, or foster parents account for the remaining 5%.

The Survey Questionnaire

We designed the survey instrument (see Appendix B) with the assistance of the CADS staff. Successive drafts of the questionnaire were sent to parents and professionals for review and suggestions. A Spanish translation of the final form of the questionnaire was arranged. Apparently this translation was flawed, resulting in more missing data in the questionnaires received from Spanish-speaking parents. The questionnaire contains seven sections:

- Background information on hearing loss, age at identification, additional conditions, hearing aids, and cochlear implants.
- Services received and level of satisfaction with services: four items based on an instrument developed by Project Dakota (used with permission of Project Dakota; see Cebe, 1996; Kovach & Jacks, 1989).
- Sources of help and degree of helpfulness, 14 items based on the Family Support Scale (used with permission from Dr. Carl Dunst [Dunst, Jenkins, & Trivette, 1984]).
- Child's behavioral characteristics, 10 items from the Meadow-Kendall Social-Emotional Assessment Inventory for Deaf and Hard of Hearing Children, Preschool Form (Meadow-Orlans, 1983, 1984).
- Child's language/communication level, 14 items adapted from the SKI*HI Language Development Scale (used with permission from SKI*HI [Tonelson & Watkins, 1979]) and from the MacArthur Communication Inventory (Fenson et al., 1991).
- Parents' response to the identification of hearing loss, nine items from the Impact of Deafness Scale (Meadow-Orlans, 1990).
- Family background characteristics.

Processing the Survey Data

Codes were constructed for 147 pieces of information from the survey questionnaire. Data were entered on a computer, and analyses were conducted using the Statistical Program for the Social Sciences (SPSS). A summary of survey results was mailed to all of the parents who had requested it, and program summaries were mailed to administrators of programs with 10 respondents or more. Tables containing detailed statistical results are included in Appendix C.

Interview Data
Telephone Interviews

Semistructured interviews (one for hearing parents and one for deaf parents) were designed to encourage parents to describe their personal experiences and to address specific issues that emerged from the data, such as the circumstances surrounding hearing loss identification, parental concerns, services provided, and advice for professionals and other parents.

We selected 40 families at random from those parents who indicated in their questionnaires a willingness for us to contact them for a telephone interview. Subsequently, 22 additional families were randomly selected from specifically identified groups, including families whose children had additional conditions, parents who were deaf or hard of hearing, parents of children with cochlear implants, and families in which one or both parents were members of minority groups.

Interviews were conducted by telephone or TTY (a telecommunications device for communicating with deaf people) and lasted between 30 and 60 minutes. Two interviews with deaf parents were conducted through an interpreter. With the permission of the parents, we tape-recorded the voice interviews and later transcribed them. TTYs printed transcripts of those interviews.

Focus Group Interviews

We conducted three focus groups with the parents of 6- and 7-year-old DF/HH children in large urban areas in order to expand the number of those families represented in the survey and telephone interview data. In preparation for this phase of the project, the three authors received formal training in leading focus groups. Parents participating in the focus groups had not completed a questionnaire; thus the focus group interview questions were similar to but more general than the individual interview questions. (A copy of the focus group interview guide appears in Appendix B). Tape-recorded discussions included comments about families' experiences, feelings, and concerns leading to the confirmation of their child's hearing loss; the people or services that were the most helpful; needs that were or were not addressed by early intervention services; the families' communication decisions; and their advice for professionals and other parents.

Coding the Interview Data

Interview responses were coded after several reviews of the interview transcripts and an inductive analysis of the data. Categories of comments were identified, and a codebook was developed. Categories were discussed and modified numerous times as the coding proceeded. Analysis was accomplished by searching for terms related to the themes that emerged during the coding process using Ethnograph, a computer-based program for qualitative data analysis that identifies segments of text using one or more code words. Forty separate code categories were identified.

These categories were used as the basis for the qualitative analyses reported in chapters 2 through 9. Transcripts were thoroughly reviewed in order to identify emerging themes, and every effort was made to include the views of parents with differing experiences and opinions. All of the names of children in interview excerpts are pseudonyms. The same code and coding process used for the telephone interviews were used for the transcribed focus group discussions.

A description of the interview coding process illustrates how the senior team functioned. One team member coded the first interview and shared her coded transcript with the other team members. A second interview was coded by all three of the team members, who discussed their codes and made additions and revisions to the codebook. The three then coded two interviews independently and compared the coded results. The team discussed these until they agreed on codebook categories and definitions. After coding three pilot interviews, the team found the coding decisions to be reliable. Two of the three senior team members independently coded the remaining transcripts in alternate pairs, comparing and discussing for coder agreement.

Limitations of the Data

Although we are fortunate to have very broad geographic and educational program coverage and even though the characteristics of the survey respondents are similar to those of children reported to Gallaudet's annual survey, the method of contacting parents does not allow for a reliable estimate of response rate to the survey. Even though proportions of non-White respondents are quite respectable, flaws in the Spanish translation may mean that the survey responses of Spanish-speaking parents are less reliable. Focus group interviews were conducted in English, so non-English-speaking parents were excluded. Finally, the numbers of parents interviewed in each subgroup are small, and interview comments cannot represent the full range of family experience. Despite these limitations we believe that the data provide a fair range of views of parents' feelings and experiences with services for themselves and their children in the first 6 or 7 years of the children's lives.

Note: Portions of this appendix are adapted from M. A. Sass-Lehrer, K. P. Meadow-Orlans, and D. M. Mertens (in press; Investigating families' experiences with early education: A team approach. In B. Bodner-Johnson & M. A. Sass-Lehrer (Eds.), *Early education for deaf and hard of hearing infants and toddlers and their families.* Baltimore: Brookes).

Letter to Parents
on Gallaudet University letterhead)

Spring 1996

To: Parents of deaf and hard of hearing children born in 1989 or 1990

From: Kay Meadow-Orlans, Gallaudet Research Institute

Donna M. Mertens, Professor, Department of Educational Foundations and Research

Marilyn Sass-Lehrer, Professor, Department of Education

We hope you will participate in our research study by completing and mailing the survey form in our self-addressed envelope within two weeks.

The purpose of the study is to learn about the kinds of services received by parents and children, how parents evaluate those services, and how parents view their child's social development and language skills.

Your participation is completely voluntary. No benefits that might be available to you would ever be withheld by Gallaudet if you choose not to participate. If you complete the survey form, we can assume that you have chosen to do so and that we have told you that you will not be placed at risk. All information is confidential. You may reply anonymously OR you may give us personal information in order to receive a copy of our report or to volunteer for a follow-up interview. If you have questions, feel free to contact Dr. Meadow-Orlans at the above address or Dr. Carolyn Corbett, Chair of the Institutional Review Board for the Protection of Human Subjects at 202-651-5540.

WE BELIEVE THAT OUR RESEARCH CAN BENEFIT PARENTS AND THEIR CHILDREN WHO ARE DEAF OR HARD OF HEARING. PLEASE HELP US TO ACHIEVE THIS GOAL.

Survey Questionnaire

GALLAUDET UNIVERSITY NATIONAL SURVEY
SUPPORT SERVICES FOR PARENTS AND THEIR DEAF OR
HARD OF HEARING CHILDREN
These questions should be answered by the adult who spends the most time with the deaf or hard of hearing child.

Relationship of respondent to child:
___ **Mother**   ___ **Father**   ___ **Other:**_____

★★★

Section I. Background Information

1. **Your child's date of birth:**

   month ____ day ____ year _____

2. **Sex:**   ___ Girl   ___ Boy

3. **Who first suspected the hearing loss?**

   ___ parent   ___ other relative

   ___ medical doctor   ___ other professional

   ___ other (who?) _____

   How old was your child then?_____

   How old was your child when a specialist CONFIRMED the diagnosis? _____

4. **What is the extent of your child's hearing loss?**

   ___ Deaf: can't understand speech, even with a hearing aid

   ___ Hard of hearing: can understand speech when in a quiet room, with a hearing aid

5. **What kinds of instruction or therapy has your child received from a teacher or specialist?**

   ___ Speech therapy: age began: _____

   ___ Auditory training: age began: _____

   ___ Sign language: age began: _____

   ___ Cued speech: age began: _____

___ Other (1) _____

age began: _____

___ Other (2) _____

age began: _____

6. Does your child have any conditions other than deafness that might affect development or education?

____ no, no other conditions

____ yes (If yes, check all that apply):

___visual impairment   ____ cerebral palsy

___brain damage   ____ epilepsy

____ health condition   ____ developmentally delayed

___behavior problem   ____ learning disability

___orthopedic condition   ____ attention deficit

___other:_____

7. Does your child have a hearing aid?

____ no   __ yes

If yes: age when first fitted with an aid:

years_____   months_____

How much does he/she wear the aid?

a. at home?   ____ always   ____ almost always

____ sometimes   ____ almost never   ____ never

b. at school?   ____ always   ____ almost always

__ sometimes   ____ almost never   ____ never

8. Has a cochlear implant been considered for your child?

____ no   ____ yes

If yes: Has he/she been evaluated for an implant?   __ no   __ yes

Was surgery performed?   ____ no   ____ yes

When?   age: years_____   months_____

Are the results satisfactory?

____ yes, very   ____ yes, somewhat   __ no

Does your child still use the implant?

____ no   __ yes

★★★

Section II. Special Services

1. **How many different special education programs did your child attend before the age of five?**_____

   In what city or county and state was the program in which your child was enrolled the longest? _____

   (state:) _____

   Child's age in that program: _____ to _____

   What communication method was used with your child there?

   ___ speech alone   ___ sign + speech

   ___ sign alone   ___ cued speech

   Did you have a program choice?   ___ yes   ___ no

   If yes: Why did you choose this program?

   If no: What kind of program might you prefer?

   _____

   _____

   _____

   Were any Deaf adults on the staff?   ___ yes   ___ no

2. **How do you evaluate that program?**

   a. The staff responded to family concerns, ideas, questions.

   ___ always   ___ often   ___ sometimes   ___ rarely

   b. The help my child received was based on his or her individual needs.

   ___ always   ___ often   ___ sometimes   ___ rarely

   c. In my meetings with staff, I was an active member of a team, not just a listener.

   ___ always   ___ often   ___ sometimes   ___ rarely

   d. Staff accepted the limit our family put on time we could devote to the program.

   ___ always   ___ often   ___ sometimes   ___ rarely

   e. I was given a choice of the communication method to be used with my child.   ___ yes   ___ no

f. My child's language progress in that program was:

___ excellent   ___ good   ___ satisfactory   ___ disappointing

3. **Please check all services available to your family since hearing loss was diagnosed:**

Information about (check all that apply):

a. ___ Deafness

b. ___ Legal rights of deaf children

c. ___ Child behavior and/or development

d. ___ Choices for future school placement

e. ___ Sign language instruction

    Received by: ___ mother   ___ father

                    ___ others (who?) _____

f. ___ Parent group meetings

    Attended by: ___ mother   ___ father

                    ___ others (who?) _____

g. ___ Individual counseling

    Received by: ___ mother   ___ father

                    ___ others (who?) _____

h. ___ Other services or instruction

    What?_____

    Received by: ___ mother   ___ father

                    ___ others (who?) _____

4. **Please circle the letter of the *one* service listed in question 3 that was MOST helpful to:**

mother   a   b   c   d   e

father   a   b   c   d   e

others   a   b   c   d   e

5. **Which method of communication is used MOST with your child *at home* NOW?**

___ speech alone   ___ cued speech

___ sign + speech   ___ sign alone

Which method of communication is used MOST with your child *at school* NOW?

___ speech alone   ___ cued speech

___ sign + speech   __ sign alone

6. What kind of school program does your child attend now?

___ Residential (day student)   ___ Residential (dorm)

___ Day school for deaf students   ___ Day school for hearing students

___ Classes with deaf students only

___ Partially mainstreamed   ___ Fully mainstreamed

★★

Section III. Sources of Help

Listed below are sources that are sometimes helpful to families with a young child. Please *circle* the response that best describes how helpful each has been to you since the diagnosis of child's hearing loss.

0 = Not at all helpful   3 = Very helpful
1 = Sometimes helpful 4 = Extremely helpful
2 = Generally helpful   NA = Not available

1. Spouse (or partner)	0	1	2	3	4	NA
2. My parents	0	1	2	3	4	NA
3. My spouse's parents	0	1	2	3	4	NA
4. My relatives	0	1	2	3	4	NA
5. My spouse's relatives	0	1	2	3	4	NA
6. My friends/spouse's friends	0	1	2	3	4	NA
7. Parents of deaf children	0	1	2	3	4	NA
8. Church (pastor, rabbi)	0	1	2	3	4	NA
9. Family doctor/pediatrician	0	1	2	3	4	NA
10. Therapist or counselor	0	1	2	3	4	NA
11. Teacher(s)/specialist(s)	0	1	2	3	4	NA

12. Deaf adults   0   1   2   3   4   NA

13. Childcare giver   0   1   2   3   4   NA

14. Other (who?)_____ 0   1   2   3   4   XX

Do you work outside the home? ____ yes ____ no

If yes: Does your employer help you meet your child's needs?

0   1   2   3   4   NA

What is your (usual) occupation?

_____

Spouse's (usual) occupation?

_____

★★★

Section IV. Your Child's Behavior

Circle the response that best describes your opinion of your child's behavior:

1 = Strongly Agree   **2 = Agree**
3 = Disagree   **4 = Strongly Disagree**

1. My child forms warm, close attachments to or friendships with peers.

   1   2   3   4

2. My child is isolated, has no friends.

   1   2   3   4

3. My child communicates with children and/or adults by any means: gesture, sign, vocalization, pantomime, speech, drawing.

   1   2   3   4

4. My child is happy, cheerful, pleasant.

   1   2   3   4

5. My child expresses concern or sympathy for others in pain or distress.

   1   2   3   4

6. My child does not express a variety of emotions appropriately (anger, fear, joy, sadness).

    1   2   3   4

7. My child has a good sense of humor and can appreciate funny situations or jokes.

    1   2   3   4

8. My child is interested in communicating with others and tries to understand them.

    1   2   3   4

9. My child forms warm, close attachments to teachers.

    1   2   3   4

10. My child initiates communication with adults.

    1   2   3   4

★★★

Section V. Questions about My Child's Language: Signed, Cued, or Spoken

1. **Does your child understand simple sentences (like "We will go to the store")?**

    ___ not yet   ___ rarely   __ sometimes   __ often

    Does your child use simple sentences?

    ___ not yet   ___ rarely   __ sometimes   __ often

2. **Does your child talk/sign about future events, for example, referring to "airplane" before you go on a trip or "swing" before you go to a park?**

    ___ not yet   ___ rarely   __ sometimes   __ often

    Does he or she most often use:

    ___ single words/signs: *airplane; swing* OR

    ___ short phrases: *airplane to grandma's; swing in park* OR

    ___ more complete sentences: *We're going on an airplane.*

3. **Does your child ask "HOW" or "WHY" questions?**

   ___ not yet   ___ rarely   ___ sometimes   ___ often

   Does he or she generally use:

   ___ single words: (*How? Why*) OR

   ___ short phrases: (*Why home?*) OR

   ___ more complete questions: (*Why are we going home?*)

4. **Does your child use sentences that express more than one idea? ("*We will go to McDonald's when Daddy comes home*")**

   ___ not yet   ___ rarely   ___ sometimes   ___ often

5. **Does your child ask serious questions, like "*What does that mean?*" or "*What happened to that boy?*"**

   ___ not yet   ___ rarely   ___ sometimes   ___ often

6. **Can your child read:**

   single words?   ___ yes   ___ no

   sentences?   ___ yes   ___ no

   story books?   ___ yes   ___ no

7. **Can your child print/write:**

   letters of the alphabet?   ___ yes   ___ no

   his/her name?   ___ yes   ___ no

   sentences?   ___ yes   ___ no

★★

Section VI. Questions about Your Own Feelings as a Parent (or Parent Substitute)

Please *circle* your response:

**1 = Strongly Agree   2 = Agree   3 = Not Sure   4 = Disagree
5 = Strongly Disagree**

1. We have more family arguments about our deaf (or hard of hearing) child than about other things.

   1   2   3   4   5

2. I feel proud of the way I have responded to the special needs of my child.

1 2 3 4 5

3. Much stress in my family is related to my child's hearing loss.

1 2 3 4 5

4. My communication skills are quite adequate for my child's needs.

1 2 3 4 5

5. Because of hearing loss, I must forget many hopes and dreams for my child.

1 2 3 4 5

6. In spite of extra time devoted to my child's needs, I still find time for myself.

1 2 3 4 5

7. My child is regularly included in family conversations because we have an effective communication system.

1 2 3 4 5

8. Parents of children with a hearing loss are expected to do too many things for them. This has been a burden for me.

1 2 3 4 5

9. There are many things I can't seem to communicate to my child.

1 2 3 4 5

★★★

Section VII. Background Questions: Family

1. **Other children in family (living at home):**

   If none, write "none."_____

   Boys: ages: ____/____/____/____/____/____

   Girls: ages: ____/____/____/____/____/____

   (**circle** the age of any child who has a hearing loss)

2. **Mother:** ___ hearing   ___ hard of hearing   ___ deaf

Father: ___ hearing   ___ hard of hearing   ___ deaf

Other: ___ hearing   ___ hard of hearing   ___ deaf

3. **With whom does child live now?**

___ mother only   ___ father only   ___ both (birth) parents

___ mother and stepfather   ___ father and stepmother

___ adoptive parent(s): age child adopted?_____

___ other: who?_____

4. **Primary language used at home:**

___ English   ___ Spanish   ___ American Sign Language

Other:_____

5. **Parents' racial or ethnic background:**

___ Whit   ___ Hispanic

___ Black/African American   ___ Native American

___ Asian/Pacific

___ Other: what?_____

6. **Are signs or cued speech used with child by:**

Mother: ___ no   ___ yes

If yes: ___ signs   ___ cued speech

Skills are: ___ excellent   ___ good   ___ fair   ___ poor

Father: ___ no   ___ yes

If yes: ___ signs   ___ cued speech

Skills are: ___ excellent   ___ good   ___ fair   ___ poor

Other: who? _____

___ no   ___ yes

If yes: ___ signs   ___ cued speech

Skills are: ___ excellent   ___ good   ___ fair   ___ poor

7. **Highest school level completed by parents:**

Mother:

___ Elementary   ___ High school

___ Vocational or secretarial

___ College (1–3 yrs)   ___ College (4 or more yrs)

Father:

___ Elementary   ___ High school

___ Vocational or secretarial

___ College (1–3 yrs)   ___ College (4 or more yrs)

★★★

THANK YOU FOR YOUR HELP WITH THIS SURVEY.

WE WELCOME YOUR COMMENTS: PLEASE ENCLOSE ANOTHER SHEET OF PAPER.

IF OUR SELF-ADDRESSED ENVELOPE IS LOST, PLEASE MAIL TO:

Dr. Kay Meadow-Orlans, Gallaudet University (KDES PAS 9), Washington, DC 20002

If you would like to receive the results of this survey, please check here ❏ and complete the mailing label below.

★★★

A small sample of those responding to the questionnaire will be selected to participate in follow-up interviews, either by phone or in person. Are you willing to be contacted for an interview?

___ No   ___ Yes

*If you would consider participating, please complete the mailing label and enter your **preferred** phone number.*

★★★

mailing label

Name _____

Street _____ Apt. _____

City & State _____ Zip _____

★★★

Preferred Phone: Day ( ) _____ - _____

                    Evening ( ) _____ -_____

[PROGRAM CODE ___ ___ - ___ ___ ___]

Interview Guides
Telephone Interviews (this was modified for parent subgroups)

Hello, may I speak to _____? This is _____ calling from Gallaudet University. I'm calling about a follow-up phone interview about support services for parents with deaf children. Last (spring) you filled out a survey for us related to support services for parents with deaf children. Do you remember that survey? I'm working with the three researchers who conducted the survey. On your survey you noted that you would be interested in a follow-up phone interview. Are you still interested in answering a few questions about support services for parents of deaf children? This interview should take about 30 minutes. Is this a good time for you to be interviewed?

First, I'll need your permission to use this conversation in our research project. Do you mind if I tape-record or (for TTY users) print the conversation for our records?

1. Can you tell me about your _____child? How would you describe him/her?

2. I see here on the survey you filled out that _____ suspected (name of child's) _____ hearing loss. Can you tell me a little bit more about that?

3. (If you need to probe, ask: "What happened next? What were your concerns? Do you know the reason for the hearing loss?")

4. What services were provided for you and your family at that time? (If there is nothing on the form, say: "I noticed that you didn't receive any services or support. Is this correct? Did you want any support services?")

5. (If services were provided, confirm the name and location of that program from the survey form.) What kind of services? Were they offered at home or in school?

6. Who or what was the most helpful to you at that time?

7. (If probing is necessary, ask: "Was there a person or program that was particularly helpful to you?")

8. I noticed from your questionnaire that you were _____ (how satisfied?) with the services that were provided at _____ (name of program). What was it about the services that did/didn't please you?

9. Are you satisfied with the school your child attends now? Why/why not?

10. Was there anything that you needed as (changed for individual parents: a deaf parent/parent of a hard of hearing child/parent of a child with a cochlear implant/parent of a child with a disability/parent of an African American, Hispanic, Asian, or other child)?

11. The next question is about communication. You indicated on your survey form that you use _____ (mode of communication). Is this right? How did you decide on this approach? Did you ever consider using other communication approaches?

12. The next two questions are about the advice you might give other people.

13. What kind of advice would you give to professionals on how to make parents like you feel more comfortable and more involved in what is going on at school? What can professionals do to motivate parents to be more involved or feel like a team member? How could professionals make parents feel more welcomed and important?

14. What kind of advice would you give to other parents who just found out that they have a child with a hearing loss?

15. Is there anything else you would like to tell me?

Thank you for your time and your help. Your responses will be very helpful to us.

Focus Group Interview Guide

1. As you introduce yourself to the group, would you tell us your first name, the name of your 6- or 7-year-old child, and something that makes you feel proud of him or her? We don't need to go around the table in turn; just speak whenever you feel like it.

2. For our first question, we'd like for you to think back to the time your child's hearing loss was first diagnosed and to describe your feelings at that time and your initial concerns.

3. Who or what was most helpful to you at that time?

4. What needs did you, your child, or other family members have that were not addressed?

5. What communication mode do you use with your child, and how were you involved in that decision?

6. What advice do you have for professionals about how to involve parents as comfortable members of an educational planning team?

7. What advice would you give to a parent whose child has just been diagnosed with a hearing loss?

Glossary and Supplementary Tables

In an effort to reduce the technical terminology and statistical information that will hold little interest for many readers of this book, we have placed almost all of the tabular data in this appendix. The tables are introduced by a glossary that provides definitions of all of the statistical tests and abbreviations in the tables.

Glossary of Statistical Terms and Abbreviations[1]

Analysis of variance (ANOVA):   A statistical technique used to test the significance of differences in the means of three or more groups.

Chi square: A statistical test to evaluate the relationship between participants' attributes on one variable (characteristic) and their attributes on another (e.g., "Do children with cochlear implants [variable/characteristic 1] have mothers who attended college [variable/characteristic 2]?").

Degrees of freedom *(df):*   The number of independent pieces of information remaining after estimating one or more parameters (values).

F: The numerical value emerging from statistical procedures performed to compute the analysis of variance test: The larger the value, the more significant the differences among the group means one is testing.

Mean *(M):*   Arithmetic average: the sum of all of the scores divided by the number of scores.

Mean square error: An estimate of the population variance in ANOVA; the denominator of the *F* ratio.

n.s.:   Not statistically significant.

---

1. Adapted from online statistical glossaries at http://www.stats.gla.ac.uk/ steps/glossary/alphabet.html and http://davidmlane.com/hyperstat/glossary.html.

Probability (*p*):   The probability that a result (here, differences between or
among groups) would occur by chance (e.g., *p* = .05, the probability that the
difference would occur by chance is 5 in 100; *p* = .01, the probability is 1 in
100; *p* = .001, the probability is 1 in 1,000). If a value is greater than .05, it is
not considered to be statistically significant ("n.s.").

Standard deviation *(sd)*:   A measure of the dispersion or variation around the
mean of a distribution of numbers. The more widely the values are spread out
(the greater the range), the larger the *sd* will be.

t: The numerical value emerging from statistical procedures performed to
compute a "*t*-test" to evaluate the differences between two means.

Table 1. Elapsed Time in Months from Confirmation of Hearing Loss to
Interventions

	All Children			Deaf			Hard of Hearing		
	Mean	SD	(N)	Mean	SD	(N)	Mean	SD	(N)
Hearing aid	7.9	11.1	(319)	8.1	12.0	(133)	7.8	10.5	(177)
Speech training	9.6	11.7	(299)	11.2	12.1	(131)	7.9	10.5	(157)
Auditory training	10.2	11.9	(272)	10.2	12.0	(116)	10.1	12.0	(149)
Sign language	11.2	13.6	(251)	10.4	13.8	(143)	11.8	13.1	(104)
Cued Speech	19.7	17.4	(48)	25.4	20.4	(19)	16.3	14.5	(28)

Table 2. Communication Approach

| | Initial Program | | | Current Program | | | Home (Currently) | | |
	All	Deaf	Hard of Hearing	All	Deaf	Hard of Hearing	All	Deaf	Hard of Hearing
Speech alone	24%	10%	38%	27%	7%	46%	33%	9%	56%
Sign + speech	66	78	54	61	75	48	56	73	41
Sign alone	5	9	1	10	17	4	10	18	3
Cued Speech	3	1	3	2	1	3	1	—	1
Signs + cues	3	2	3	—	1	—	—	1	—
Total	101	100	99	100	101	101	100	101	101
(N)	(360)	(173)	(176)	(383)	(176)	(193)	(384)	(176)	(194)

Table 3. Parents' Evaluations of Early Services

	Always	Often	Sometimes	Rarely	(N)
The staff responded to family concerns, ideas, and questions.	74%	18%	7%	2%	(367)
The help my child received was based on his or her individual needs.	69	22	8	2	(369)
In my meetings with staff, I was an active listener.	64	20	11	5	(366)
Staff accepted the limit our family put on the time we could devote to the program.	65	22	11	3	(352)

Table 4. Program Evaluation Scores by Mothers' Hearing Status and by Racial/Ethnic Background

	Mean	SD	(N)
Mother's hearing status[1]			
Hearing	14.28	2.37	(302)
Deaf/hard of hearing	12.63	3.34	(32)
Racial/ethnic background[2]			
White	14.26	2.47	(250)
Non-White/mixed race	13.66	2.74	(114)

[1] $t (34.39) = -2.73; p = .01$

[2] $t (362) = -2.10; p < .04$

Table 5. Sources of Help for Parents: Evaluations of Degree of Helpfulness (Mean Ratings, Scale = 0–4)★

Help Source	Mean	SD	(N)
Teacher	3.52	.78	(368)
Spouse	2.88	1.33	(330)
Therapist	2.68	1.31	(236)
Other parents	2.64	1.31	(281)
Deaf adults	2.56	1.35	(218)
Own parents	2.53	1.41	(320)
Child's caregiver	2.34	1.43	(198)
Friends	2.16	1.25	(334)
Own relatives	2.14	1.35	(326)
Doctor/pediatrician	2.09	1.31	(337)
Spouse's parents	1.82	1.43	(284)
Spouse's relatives	1.67	1.40	(266)
Church (pastor, rabbi)	1.65	1.43	(224)

Note: Only 24 respondents checked "Other" and named an additional help source.

★0 = not at all helpful; 1 = sometimes helpful; 2 = generally helpful; 3 = very helpful; 4 = extremely helpful

Table 6. Mean Support Index★ by Racial/Ethnic Background and by Mothers' Educational Level with ANOVA Summary

Mother's Education	White	Non-White/Mixed
Some college	25.32	24.51
(N)	(158)	(55)
No college	23.78	19.83
(N)	(101)	(54)

Analysis of Variance (ANOVA)			
	df	F	p
Race	1	5.086	<.05
Education	1	5.766	<.05
Race by Education	1	1.936	n.s.
Error	364	(96.22 = mean square error)	

★A support index was created by dividing the sum of responses to items shown in Table 5 by the total number of help sources available. Overall mean (N = 372) = 23.9 (SD = 9.92); range = 2–52.

Table 7. Children's Mean Behavior Item Scores (SD)

Characteristic	All Children	Children With Problems	Children Without Problems	t-values
Initiates conversations/adults	3.25 (.83)	2.88 (.78)	3.29 (.82)	2.76**
Forms close friendships/peers	3.31 (.73)	2.94 (.69)	3.36 (.72)	3.35**
Empathizes w/pain, distress	3.37 (.83)	2.88 (.88)	3.42 (.80)	3.67***
Expresses range of emotions	3.39 (.89)	2.85 (1.12)	3.43 (.85)	2.91**
Has good sense of humor	3.47 (.74)	3.27 (.76)	3.50 (.73)	1.66
Close attachments/teachers	3.48 (.68)	3.09 (.78)	3.52 (.65)	3.47***
Communicates, any means	3.48 (.78)	3.38 (.70)	3.49 (.78)	.76
Not isolated, has friends	3.51 (.75)	2.94 (1.01)	2.56 (.71)	3.49***
Interested in communication	3.53 (.70)	3.26 (.67)	3.56 (.68)	2.44*
Happy, cheerful, pleasant	3.55 (.64)	3.15 (.51)	3.59 (.63)	4.66***
Total score	3.42 (.51)	3.08 (.48)	3.47 (.50)	4.36***

Note: All children, $N = 393$; children with behavior problems, $N = 34$; children without behavioral problems, $N = 349$.

$*p \leq .05$; $**p \leq .01$; $***p \leq .001$

Table 8. Mean Behavior Scores by Child's Hearing Level, Age at Identification (Above and Below Median for Hearing Level Group), and Additional Conditions with ANOVA Summary

Age at Identification	Deaf		Hard of Hearing	
	Early	Late	Early	Late
Additional Conditions:				
None	3.62	3.55	3.56	3.20
(N)	(60)	(61)	(71)	(56)
One or more	3.20	3.26	3.28	3.48
(N)	(30)	(16)	(36)	(28)

Analysis of Variance (ANOVA)			
	df	F	p
Additional conditions	1	10.468	≤.001
Identification/Hearing Loss	3	2.921	≤.05
Additional Conditions by Identification and Hearing Loss	3	7.680	≤.001
Error	350	(.40 = mean square error)	

Table 9. Mean Behavior Scores by Racial/Ethnic Background, and by Mother's Education with ANOVA Summary

Mother	White	Non-White/Mixed
Some college	3.46	3.52
(N)	(166)	(57)
No college	3.45	3.23
(N)	(102)	(57)

Analysis of Variance (ANOVA)			
	df	F	p
Race	1	2.168	n.s.
Education	1	3.364	n.s.
Race by Education	1	5.983	≤.05
Error	364	(.26 = mean square error)	

Table 10. Children's Performance on Individual Language Items: Proportion Achieving Highest Rating

	Percent	(N)
Understands simple sentences "often"	77%	(399)
Uses simple sentences "often"	64	(397)
Talks/signs about future events "often"	66	(393)
. . . using more complete sentences	46	(393)
Asks *how* or *why* questions "often"	58	(398)
. . . using "more complete questions"	42	(386)
Uses sentences expressing more than one idea "often"	43	(397)
Asks serious questions (e.g., "What does that mean?") "often"	48	(399)
Child can read:		
Single words	80	(387)
Sentences	46	(389)
Books	35	(389)
Child can print/write:		
Letters of the alphabet	91	(390)
His/her name	93	(390)
Sentences	43	(390)

Table 11. Mean Language Scores★ by Child's Hearing Level, Age at Identification Early or Late (Above vs. Below Median for Hearing Level Group), and Presence of Additional Conditions with ANOVA Summary

	Deaf		Hard of Hearing	
Age at Identification	Early	Late	Early	Late
Additional Conditions:				
None	30.04	30.91	33.46	31.68
(N)	(57)	(58)	(74)	(56)
One or more	22.93	27.06	25.94	30.21
(N)	(29)	(16)	(36)	(28)

Analysis of Variance (ANOVA)			
	df	F	p
Additional conditions	1	25.71	≤.001
Identification/Hearing Loss	3	2.93	≤.05
Additional Conditions by Identification and Hearing Loss	3	1.99	n.s.
Error	346	(80.90 = mean square error)	

★Parents assessed their child's usage of items shown in Table 10 as "not yet," "rarely," "sometimes," or "often" (assigned scores of 0, 1, 2, or 3) for spoken/signed items, and "yes" or "no" (assigned scores of 0 or 3) for items on reading and writing. This procedure yielded a language score ranging from 0 to 42 points, with a mean, based on the scores for 390 children, of 29.8 (SD = 9.8).

Table 12. Mean Language Scores by Racial/Ethnic Background and by Mother's Educational Level with ANOVA Summary

Mother's Education	White	Non-White/Mixed
Some college	32.28	28.56
(N)	(159)	(59)
No college	28.95	26.03
(N)	(100)	(66)

Analysis of Variance (ANOVA)		
	df	F	p
Race	1	13.46	≤.001.
Education	1	9.66	≤.01
Race by Education| 1	.15	n.s.
Error	382	(90.01 = mean square error)	

Table 13. Impact of Deafness on Parents and Families
(Mean Scores, Scale 1–5)★

Scale Item	Mean
There are many things I can't seem to communicate to my child.	3.48
Much stress in my family is related to hearing loss.	3.73
In spite of extra time devoted to child's needs, I still find time for myself.	3.74
My communication skills are quite adequate for my child's needs.	3.79
My child is regularly included in family conversations because we have an effective communication system.	4.02
We have more family arguments about our deaf (or hard of hearing child than about other things.)	4.20
Parents of children with a hearing loss are expected to do too many things for them. This has been a burden to me.	4.25
I feel proud of the way I have responded to the special needs of my child.	4.46
Because of my child's hearing loss, I must forget many hopes and dreams for him or her.	4.56

★ 1 = strongly agree; 2 = agree; 3 = not sure; 4 = disagree; 5 = strongly disagree
Mean Impact score for all nine items = 4.02, SD = .63.

with Jennifer Pittaway

Books, Videos, and CD-ROMs

A Basic Course in American Sign Language (Un Curso Basico de Lenguaje Americano de Señas)*

Tom Humphries, Carol Padden, and Terence J. O'Rourke. Translated by Lourdes Rubio.

Silver Spring, MD: TJ, 1991; 2nd edition 1994

ISBN 0-93266-643-4 (hardcover); 0-93266-642-6 (paperback)

This book features nearly 1,000 vocabulary items, illustrations, brief explanations, and examples of some of the basic structures of American Sign Language. It includes exercises for student practice. (The translation features English and Spanish side by side.)

But What about My Deaf Child?

Virginia Duncan

York, PA: Parent Education Network, 1997

A guidebook for parents of deaf or hard of hearing children to assist them in understanding their rights and developing a strong network of support and resources for their child. Designed for parents and caregivers in Pennsylvania, this book addresses evaluation, the IFSP/IEP process, services, communication, placement issues, and conflict resolution. Appendices include descriptions of communication methods, checklists

---

*Sources of special interest to minority parents
**Sources of special interest to parents of children with additional conditions

for the IFSP or IEP meetings, and names of professional organizations and other resources for parents.

Choices in Deafness: A Parent's Guide to Communication Options

Sue Schwartz, Ed.
Bethesda, MD: Woodbine House, 1996; 2nd edition
ISBN 0-933149-85-9
This text is useful for learning about the communication options open to a child with a hearing loss. The approaches include auditory verbal, bilingual-bicultural, Cued Speech, oral, and Total Communication. This edition explains the medical causes of hearing loss, the diagnostic process, audiological assessment, and cochlear implants. Children and parents describe their personal experiences. Glossary; reading and resource lists.

Cochlear Implantation for Infants and Children

Graeme M. Clark, Robert S. Cowan, and Richard C. Dowell
San Diego: Singular, 1997
ISBN 1-5659-3727-9
This book presents the surgical, medical, audiological, speech and language, and habilitation aspects of cochlear implantation in infants and children. Drawn from a body of research about the clinical management of children with cochlear implants, the book describes the criteria for acceptance as a cochlear implant candidate and different habilitation techniques. Authors discuss approaches to implanting infants and patients with more residual hearing.

Cochlear Implants: A Handbook

Bonnie Poitras Tucker
Jefferson, NC: McFarland, 1998
ISBN 0-7864-0534-1
This book explains how cochlear implants work, for whom they work, and the extent to which deaf people benefit. The author tells of her own experience with an implant and provides a history of cochlear implants.

Questionnaire responses, summaries, case studies, and general information from experts in the field detail the feelings of implant recipients and their families.

Cochlear Implants for Kids

Warren Estabrooks, Ed.
Washington, DC: Alexander Graham Bell Association, 1998
ISBN 0-8820-0208-2
Designed to educate readers about cochlear implants, including surgery, the importance of rehabilitation, and the significance of parents' and professionals' roles, this 404-page book also includes trained professionals' diverse approaches to therapy, as well as parents' personal narratives.

Cochlear Implants in Children: Ethics and Choices

John B. Christiansen and Irene W. Leigh
Washington, DC: Gallaudet University Press, 2002
ISBN 1-56368-116-1
This book covers the ongoing controversy about implanting cochlear hearing devices in children. It describes findings from a survey and follow-up interviews with parents of children who have implants. It also includes a history of implants and an explanation of how they work, as well as parents' reports of how they learned about implants and selected an implant center and their children's experiences and progress.

Come Sign with Us: Sign Language Activities for Children*

Jan C. Hafer and Robert M. Wilson
Washington, DC: Gallaudet University Press, 1996; 2nd edition
ISBN 1-56368-051-3
An illustrated activities manual for teaching children sign language, this book features more than 300 line drawings of people signing familiar words, phrases, and sentences using ASL signs in English word order. Equivalent words are listed in both English and Spanish. Includes

supplemental information about deafness, the origins of ASL, and the Deaf community.

Deaf Children, Their Families, and Professionals: Dismantling Barriers

Sarah Beazley and Michael Moore
London: David Fulton, 1995
ISBN 1-85346-354-X

This book aims to reduce the "disablement" of children and their families. It focuses on deaf children and combines families' recommendations with discussions about the avoidance of disability barriers.

Deaf Like Me

Thomas Spradley and James P. Spradley
Washington, DC: Gallaudet University Press, 1997
ISBN 0-930323-11-4

This book details the Spradley family's efforts to provide communication for a deaf daughter after they are advised that oralism is "the only way to go." This updated version includes an epilogue by the daughter, describing her experiences growing up deaf and her struggle to communicate.

Deaf Plus: A Multicultural Perspective*

Kathee Christensen, Ed.
Berkeley: DawnSignPress, 2000
ISBN 1-58121-017-5

Teachers, administrators, psychologists, social workers, and families with deaf children will learn much from these 11 essays about the multilingual and multicultural dimensions of the Deaf community. Included are a historical overview of multicultural education programs for deaf students, schooling, and family involvement for children from diverse backgrounds, and the educational and social needs of deaf children with a Spanish-speaking heritage: Hispanic, Latino, or Chicano. The book presents recommendations for educational reform to facilitate increased dialogue, research, and practice to meet the cultural and linguistic needs of deaf children.

Educational and Communication Needs of Deaf and Hard of Hearing Children: A Statement of Principle Regarding Fundamental Systemic Educational Change

Lawrence Siegel
National Deaf Education Project, 2000
300 Drakes' Landing, Suite 172
Greenbrae, CA 94904

The statement of principle proposes educational reform to provide deaf and hard of hearing children with a language-rich educational experience. It describes the need to provide educational programming that fosters age-appropriate language skills in classrooms that are fully available with a critical mass of communication peers and where staff can communicate effectively.

Educational Intervention for the Student with Multiple Disabilities**

Donna Irons-Reavis
Springfield, IL: C. C. Thomas, 1992
ISBN 0-39805-793-1

This book includes material on life skills, teacher training, and classroom techniques for deaf children with additional conditions.

El Jardin Silencisoso: Criando a su Hijo Sordo*

Paul Ogden
Hillsboro, OR: Butte, 2002
ISBN 1-884362-56-7

This Spanish translation of the first five chapters of Paul Ogden's *The Silent Garden* provides guidance to Spanish-speaking parents of deaf children. These chapters emphasize two foundational themes: (1) for a successful life, deaf children need a positive experience with their families and (2) the central issue of deafness is communication instead of hearing loss.

Facilitating Hearing and Listening in Young Children

Carol Flexer
San Diego: Singular, 1999; 2nd edition
ISBN 1-5659-3989-1
Emphasizing the need to create an "auditory world," this book presents information on many facets of hearing loss, amplification technology, cochlear implants, federal laws, and listening strategies.

Families with Deaf Children: Discovering Your Needs and Exploring Your Choices

VHS videocassette
Boys Town, NE: Boys Town Press, 1996
ISBN 0-93851-083-5
This videocassette is a guide to the difficult choices that confront parents of deaf children. The parents in this videotape have different feelings and make different choices, but all of them see their children as young people who can succeed in their families and communities. The stories provide a starting point for discussion and decision making.

Families with Hard of Hearing Children: What If Your Child Has a Hearing Loss?

VHS videocassette
Boys Town, NE: Boys Town Press, 1996
ISBN 0-938510-80-0
This video helps parents of children with a partial hearing loss know what's ahead. Following two families in their search for answers, the tape provides useful guidance about working with audiologists and school personnel to meet these children's needs. It shows parents that hard of hearing children can lead normal lives and get along well with peers.

A Family's Guide to the Individualized Family Services Plan

Juliann J. Woods Cripe
VHS videocassette
Baltimore: Paul H. Brookes, 1995
ISBN 1-55766-220-7

Designed to assist in navigating the Individualized Family Service Plan (IFSP) process, this video outlines the roles of professionals; describes what happens during an IFSP meeting; discusses legislation relevant to the IFSP; and explains how to document a child's services, resources, and desired outcomes.

The Hearing Aid Handbook: User's Guide for Children

Donna S. Wayner
Washington, DC: Gallaudet University Press, 1990
ISBN 0-9303-2373-4

A brief (50-page) illustrated book encouraging children's use of hearing aids.

HyperSign: An Interactive Dictionary of American Sign Language*

Doug Martin and Anne Lieberth
CD-ROM and videocassette
Campton, NH: Trinity Software, 1997
ISBN 0-92736-553-7

An ASL dictionary that contains more than 2,000 words that one can search by name or category or by simply scrolling to the word. Full-motion video illustrates each word. The dictionary can be set for use by a child, teen, or adult and in English or Spanish.
Internet: http://www.trinitysoftware.com/speech/index.html

IDEA Advocacy for Children Who Are Deaf or Hard of Hearing: A Question-and-Answer Book for Parents and Professionals

Bonnie P. Tucker
San Diego: Singular Publishing Group, 1997
ISBN 1-56593-896-8
This book aims to empower parents of children with a hearing loss to obtain the appropriate educational services that the 1997 Individuals with Disabilities Education Act (IDEA) mandated.

Issues in Deaf Education

Susan Gregory, Stephen Powers, Linda Watson, Pamela Knight, and Wendy McCracken, Eds.
London: David Fulton, 1998
ISBN 1-85346-512-7
This book offers a comprehensive review of recent research and current issues in educational policy, psychology, linguistics, and audiology as they relate to the education of deaf children. It includes suggestions for additional reading.

Keys to Raising a Deaf Child

V. Frazier-Maiwald and L. M. Williams
New York: Barron's, 1999
ISBN 0-76410-723-2
Discussion begins with the child and family and then moves to collaborations with others outside the home (medical professionals, the Deaf community, educators, schools, and audiologists). This book is designed to help parents make choices about communication and language. The last sections focus on language, suggesting bimodal (sign language as well as speech) strategies for the home, building language socially and academically, and linking language and literacy. As educators, the authors (one of whom is the parent of two deaf children) offer practical suggestions and support for parents.

Kid-Friendly Parenting with Deaf and Hard of Hearing Children

Daria J. Medwid and Denise Chapman Weston
Washington, DC: Laurent Clerc National Deaf Education Center, Gallaudet University Press, 1995
ISBN 1-56368-031-9

This step-by-step guide offers ideas and methods for children ages 3 to 12. It provides play activities to enhance communication, solve problems, and strengthen relationships. The book presents techniques for setting limits while avoiding power struggles and fostering behavior changes. Included is information about special resources and support services.

Mi Nombre Es Lupita y Tengo un Hijo Sordo (My Name Is Lupita and I Have a Deaf Son)*

Gina Aguirre-Larson
Hillsboro, OR: Butte, 1996
ISBN 1-88436-216-8

These six Spanish booklets not only introduce parents to essential information but are also useful for professionals who work with Spanish-speaking families. Topics include parts and functions of the ear; types, causes, and degrees of hearing loss; testing; audiology; hearing aids and cochlear implants; language and social development; communication and education philosophies; and home activities for language development.

Negotiating the Special Education Maze: A Guide for Parents and Teachers*

Winifred Anderson, Stephen Chitwood, and Deidre Hayden
Bethesda, MD: Woodbine House, 1997; 3rd edition
ISBN 0-93314-972-7

This is a practical, step-by-step guide for parents of children with special needs and the teachers and professionals who assist them. Designed to help parents to be effective advocates and decision makers, the book explains how school systems work, what services are available, and what rights and benefits the Individuals with Disabilities Education Act and related federal laws provide. The guide has personalized checklists, exercises, and charts to help parents obtain appropriate services for their child. Available in Spanish.

The New Language of Toys: Teaching Communication Skills to Children with Special Needs: A Guide for Parents and Teachers

Sue Schwartz and Joan E. Heller Miller
Bethesda, MD: Woodbine House, 1996; revised edition
ISBN 0-933149-73-5
With suggestions for using everyday toys, this book presents a hands-on approach to developing communication skills in children with disabilities. It describes a wide assortment of toys and books for children ranging from birth through age 6 years. Included are chapters on computer technology, language learning, videotapes, and television.

Not Deaf Enough: Raising a Child Who Is Hard of Hearing with Hugs, Humor, and Imagination

Patricia Ann Morgan Candlish
Washington, DC: Alexander Graham Bell Association for the Deaf, 1996
ISBN 0-8820-0201-5
This book portrays a family's struggle to identify, accept, and support their youngest child and the diagnosis of his mild-to-moderate hearing loss. With great detail and frankness, the mother describes the challenges the entire family faces. They come together to grieve and then to cope with the hearing loss. A parent's perspective provides an overview of services for hard of hearing children.

Raising and Educating a Deaf Child

Marc Marschark
New York: Oxford University Press, 1997
ISBN 0-19-509467-0
This is a comprehensive guide to raising a deaf or hard of hearing child. It covers medical causes of early hearing loss, language acquisition, social

and intellectual development, education, and environment. Researchers, educators, students and parents will find helpful the detailed information about the impact of hearing loss on development. Included is a list of information sources and organizations for deaf children.

Reading to Deaf Children: Learning from Deaf Adults*

David R. Schleper
Manual and VHS videocassettes
Washington, DC: Laurent Clerc National Deaf Education Center, Gallaudet University, 1995
This title describes and demonstrates 15 research-based principles from studies of deaf parents and teachers who are effective storybook readers. The manual has been translated into six other languages: Arabic, Chinese, Russian, Spanish, Tagalog, and Vietnamese; the accompanying videotape is dubbed in the same language as the manual.

The Signing Family: What Every Parent Should Know about Sign Communication

David A. Stewart and Barbara Luetke-Stahlman
Washington, DC: Gallaudet University Press, 1998
ISBN 1-56368-069-6
This book describes and supports the visual-gestural nature of signing. Chapters describe major signing options, such as American Sign Language, Signed English, Signing Exact English, and Contact Sign.

Signing Fiesta*

Connie Salvador and Merced Gonzalez
VHS videocassettes
Santa Maria, CA: New Rule Productions, 1996
These eleven videos are signed in ASL with voice-over in Spanish and English. They contain stories, elementary sentences, and hundreds of signs related to family, school, and hearing loss. Vocabulary includes animals, insects, school, colors, family, festivities, action verbs, food, feelings, and questions.
Internet: http://members.aol.com/signfiesta/index.htm

Signs for Me*

Ben Bahan and Joe Dannis
Berkeley: DawnSignPress, 1990
ISBN 0915035278
Designed for preschool and elementary children, this vocabulary book has captioned pictures with sign illustrations. Included are the manual alphabet, number signs, and different ASL handshapes. The index is in eight languages, including Spanish, Hmong, and Vietnamese.

The Silent Garden: Raising Your Deaf Child

Paul Ogden
Washington, DC: Gallaudet University Press, 1996; 2nd edition
ISBN 1-5636-8058-0
This introductory guide for parents was written by a deaf author. Topics include types of hearing loss, communication options, school environments, professional help, and technological aids. Case studies, interviews with parents, and an index of resources provide additional information.

So Your Child Has a Hearing Loss: Next Steps for Parents

Susan Coffmann
Alexander Graham Bell Association for the Deaf and Hard of Hearing, 2000 (AG Bell)
This 32-page booklet addresses the selection of a communication method, educational decisions, and hearing technologies (hearing aids, cochlear implants, and assistive listening devices). Single copies are available free of charge; the booklet can also be purchased in bulk.
AG Bell's Publication Sales Department: Tel.: 202-337-5220 Voice; Tel.: 202-337-5221 TTY

Speak to Me!

Marcia Calhoun Forecki
Washington, DC: Gallaudet University Press, 1985
ISBN 0-930323-68-8

This is an account of the author's life with Charlie, a deaf 7-year-old. It recounts her struggle as a single parent to care for her child, find the right schools, and establish communication with her son.

Strategies for Working with Families of Young Children with Disabilities**

Paula J. Beckman, Ed.
Baltimore: Paul H. Brookes, 1996
ISBN 1-55766-257-6
This book offers techniques for collaborating with and supporting families with young children who have a disability. Focused on appropriate program planning and implementation, specific issues for early intervention specialists are addressed, such as cultural diversity, transitions to new programs, and disagreements between families and professionals.

That's My Child: Strategies for Parents of Children with Disabilities**

Lizanne Capper
Washington, DC: Child and Family Press, 1996
ISBN 0-87868-595-2
This book explores the different sources of support available to parents with children with all types of disabilities. It surveys school systems, physicians, therapists, and support organizations, as well as parents of special needs children, friends, and family—all wanting the best for these children.

You and Your Deaf Child: A Self-Instructional Guide for Parents of Deaf and Hard of Hearing Children

John Adams
Washington, DC: Laurent Clerc National Deaf Education Center, Gallaudet University, 1997; 2nd edition
ISBN 1-56368-060-2
Eleven chapters focus on topics such as feelings about hearing loss, differences in language development, and effective behavior management.

Many chapters contain practice activities and questions to help parents retain skills and evaluate their grasp of the material. The final chapter provides references and a general resource list for parents.

When Your Child Has a Disability: The Complete Sourcebook of Daily and Medical Care**

Mark L. Batshaw, Ed.
Baltimore: Paul H. Brookes, 2001; revised edition
ISBN 1-55766-472-2
This book offers practical information and direct answers to families' questions. It presents detailed coverage of specific disabilities: mental retardation, autism, hearing impairment, Down syndrome, visual impairment, communication disorders, seizure disorders, spina bifida, ADHD, cerebral palsy, and genetic syndromes. New to this edition are chapters on nutrition, dental care, legal rights and benefits, and the transition to adulthood, as well as information on development and commonly used medications. The book addresses common parent concerns such as sleep, behavior, medication, and potential complications.

El Lenguaje por Señas Simplificade (Sign Language Made Simple)*

Edgar D. Lawrence
Springfield, MO: Gospel, 1992
ISBN 0-88243-300-8
This book includes a history of sign language and a chapter on religion for deaf children as well as sign language instruction.

Organizations and Support Groups

Alexander Graham Bell Association for the Deaf and Hard of Hearing, Inc. (AG Bell)

3417 Volta Place NW
Washington, DC 20007

Tel.: 202-337-5220 Voice/TDD
Internet: http://www.agbell.org
Gathers and disseminates information on hearing loss. Promotes the early detection of hearing loss in infants. Encourages the use of speech and speechreading.

American Society for Deaf Children (ASDC)

Box 3355
Gettysburg, PA 17325
Tel.: 800-942-ASDC Voice/TTY Parent Hotline
Internet: http://www.deafchildren.org
A national organization for families and professionals. Advocates for high-quality programs and services for children and their families. Promotes meaningful and full communication access for deaf children.

Auditory-Verbal International (AVI)

2121 Eisenhower Avenue, Suite 402
Alexandria, VA 22314
Tel.: 703-739-1049 Voice; Tel.: 703-739-0874 TDD
Internet: http://www.auditory-verbal.org
Promotes listening and speaking for deaf and hard of hearing children. Supports quality educational opportunities for parents and professionals to enable children to be educated in regular classrooms.

The Children's Institute

6301 Northumberland Street
Pittsburgh, PA 15217
Tel.: 412-420-2400
Internet: http://www.amazingkids.org
Promotes the well-being of children, young people, and their families and the provision of services that meet their special needs.

Cochlear Implant Association, Inc. (CIAI)

5335 Wisconsin Avenue, NW, Suite 440
Washington, DC 20015-2052

Tel.: 202-895-2781 Voice/TTY
Internet: http://www.cici.org
A nonprofit organization that provides support, information, and access to local support groups for adults and children who have cochlear implants. Advocates for the rights and services for people with hearing loss. Formerly known as Cochlear Implant Club International.

Deaf Education Website

Internet: http://www.deafed.net
A comprehensive website designed to support the preparation of new teachers, provide resources and opportunities to deaf students, and increase collaborative activities among individuals involved in deaf education. The website provides information on upcoming events, a bulletin board for open forums and discussions, cyber mentoring, and links to professional organizations, publications, and resources.

Families for Hands and Voices

Box 371926
Denver, CO 80237
Tel.: 866-422-0422 (toll free)
Internet: http://handsandvoices.org/index.html
A parent-driven, nonprofit organization dedicated to providing unbiased support to families with children who are deaf or hard of hearing. Support activities include outreach events, educational seminars, advocacy, lobbying efforts, parent-to-parent networking, and a newsletter.

Intertribal Deaf Council*

Internet: http://deafnative.com
Upholds and continues the Native American traditions and holds events and conventions for Native American deaf and hard of hearing people in the United States and Canada.

John Tracy Clinic

806 W. Adams Boulevard
Los Angeles, CA 90007

Tel.: 800-522-4582 Voice/TTY

Internet: http://www.jtc.org

Provides worldwide parent-centered services to young children with a hearing loss and guidance for families. Promotes early identification, early intervention, and parent support and education. Promotes spoken language for deaf children. Information is available in Spanish.

Laurent Clerc National Deaf Education Center

Dean Katherine A. Jankowski

800 Florida Avenue NE

Washington, DC 20002

Tel.: 202-651-5031 Voice/TTY; Tel.: 202-651-5109

Internet: http://clerccenter.gallaudet.edu

Laurent Clerc National Deaf Education Center at Gallaudet University develops, evaluates, and disseminates innovative curricula, instructional techniques, strategies, and materials, with the aim of improving the quality of education for deaf and hard of hearing children and youth from birth through age 21 years. It is composed of Kendall Demonstration Elementary School, Model Secondary School for the Deaf, Exemplary Programs and Research, Training and Professional Development, Publications and Information Dissemination, and Information Systems and Computer Support.

The Listen-Up Listserv

Internet: http://www.listen-up.org.

Supports the informational and emotional needs of parents of deaf children with varying degrees of hearing loss and using different communication methods.

National Association of the Deaf (NAD)

814 Thayer Avenue

Silver Spring, MD 20910-4500

Tel.: 301-587-1788 Voice; Tel.: 301-587-1789 TTY

Internet: http://www.nad.org

The oldest and largest constituency organization of deaf and hard of hearing Americans in education, employment, healthcare, and communications.

National Black Deaf Advocates (NBDA)*

246 Sycamore Street, Suite 100
Decatur, GA 30030
Tel.: 404-687-9155 TTY; Tel.: 404-687-8290 Voice
Internet: http://www.nbda.org
Promotes the well-being, culture, and empowerment of African Americans who are deaf or hard of hearing. NBDA strives to strengthen the educational, cultural, social, and economic advancement of deaf and hard of hearing African Americans.

National Cued Speech Association (NCSA)

Information Service
23970 Hermitage Road
Shaker Heights, OH 44122
Tel.: 800-459-3529 Voice/TTY
Internet: http://www.cuedspeech.org
Promotes and supports the effective use of Cued Speech. Provides educational services, establishes standards for Cued Speech, and certifies Cued Speech instructors and transliterators.

National Deaf Education Project

Lawrence M. Siegel, Director
Tel.: 415-925-6798 TTY; Tel.: 415-925-6797
E-mail: NDEP@worldnet.att.net
A collaborative project of the American Society for Deaf Children, the Conference of Educational Administrators of Schools for the Deaf, the Convention of American Instructors of the Deaf, Gallaudet University, the National Association of the Deaf, and the National Technical Institute of the Deaf. Established in 1998 to reform the educational delivery system for deaf and hard of hearing children. Goals are to create an educational paradigm that is communication driven and to assist professional, con-

sumer, and parent organizations in addressing local, regional, and state issues affecting deaf and hard of hearing children.

National Deaf Latinas/Latinos*

Deaf Aztlán
Box 14431
San Francisco, CA 94114
Internet: http://www.deafvision.net/aztlan
Promotes the well-being, culture, and empowerment of Latinas and Latinos who are deaf or hard of hearing. Deaf Aztlán is an online resource for those living in the United States. In addition to this website, a news and discussion list is available.

National Information Center for Children and Youth with Disabilities* ** (NICHCY)

Box 1492
Washington, DC 20013-1492
Tel.: 800-695-0285 Voice/TTY; Tel.: 202-884-8200 Voice/TTY
Internet: http://www.nichcy.org
NICHCY provides fact sheets, state resource sheets, and general information to assist parents, educators, caregivers, advocates, and others in helping children and youth with disabilities participate as fully as possible at school, at home, and in their community. Many of NICHCY's publications are available in Spanish, and all of them are available on the Internet.

Self-Help for Hard of Hearing People, Inc. (SHHH)

7910 Woodmont Avenue, Suite 1200
Bethesda, MD 20814
Tel.: 301-657-2248 Voice; Tel.: 301-657-2249 TTY
Internet: http://www.shhh.org
Represents consumers who are hard of hearing and advocates for enhancing the quality of life for all people who are hard of hearing.

Beach Center on Disability: Family Resources**

The University of Kansas
Haworth Hall, Room 3136
1200 Sunnyside Avenue
Lawrence, KS 66045-7534
Tel.: 785-864-7600
Internet: http://www.beachcenter.org
The central mission of the Beach Center on Disability is to enhance the quality of life of families and their children with disabilities.

Boys Town National Research Hospital

555 North 30th Street
Omaha, NE 68131
Internet: http://www.boystownhospital.org/parents/info/index.asp
Internet: http://www.babyhearing.org
Provides a variety of helpful information and support related to hearing loss in children. Website provides information for families and professionals about newborn hearing screening and guidance for families as they take the "next steps."

KidsWorld Deaf Net (KWDN)

Internet: http://clerccenter2.gallaudet.edu/KidsWorldDeafNet
KidsWorld Deaf Net, a national communication network for parents and professionals involved in the education of deaf children, sponsored by the Laurent Clerc National Deaf Education Center with support from the AT&T Foundation, is a national communication network with information for professionals and parents. It includes both a virtual library with e-documents and useful links and a discussion forum area that includes live chats with the e-document authors and a forum for continued dialogue.

Marion Downs National Center for Infant Hearing

Internet: http://www.Colorado.edu/slhs/mdnc
Committed to establishing early hearing detection and intervention; emphasizes parent and consumer group involvement and provides coordi-

nation of statewide systems for screening, diagnosis, and intervention for newborns and infants with hearing loss.

MUMS: National Parent-to-Parent Network**

Internet: http://www.netnet.net/mums
Connect to other parents and find out about services for a child with a disability.

National Center for Hearing Assessment and Management (NCHAM)

Internet: www.infanthearing.org
Established at Utah State University to ensure that all infants and toddlers with a hearing loss are identified as early as possible and provided with timely and appropriate audiological, educational, and medical intervention. Since 1995, NCHAM has been instrumental in helping hospitals and states across the country implement Early Hearing Detection and Intervention (EHDI) programs. The website includes information on early hearing detection, intervention, and resources, including newborn hearing screening, diagnostic audiology, legislation, family support, and program evaluation.

National Deaf Education Network and Clearinghouse

Tel.: 202-651-5051 Voice; Tel.: 202-651-5052 TTY
Internet: http://clerccenter.gallaudet.edu/infotogo
Info to Go, formerly the National Information Center on Deafness, is a centralized source of up-to-date information on deafness and hearing loss in ages 0–21 years. Responds to a wide range of questions from the general public, deaf and hard of hearing people, their families, and professionals who work with them.

Our-Kids**

Internet: http://www.our-kids.org
A listserv devoted to providing support for parents, caregivers, and others working with children with special needs.

Resources for Black Deaf People*

Internet: http://www.deafweb.org/blackdef.htm

Resources for Hispanic Deaf and Hard of Hearing Populations*

Internet: http://clerccenter.gallaudet.edu/infotogo/hispanic.html

Virtual Tour of the Ear

Contains illustrations and explanations of the various parts of the ear in layperson's terms.
Internet: http://www.augie.edu/perry/ear/ear.htm

Where Do We Go from Hear?*

Internet: http://www.gohear.org
Created by parents of deaf and hard of hearing children to "provide information for families of infants and children diagnosed with a hearing loss and the professionals who work with these individuals." The web-based bibliography is organized into three broad categories: general multicultural and multilingual resource materials; multicultural and multilingual materials that reference specific cultural or linguistic deaf individuals or groups; and multicultural and multilingual materials that focus on interpreters or interpreting. Resources focus on four major target groups: African American/Black; Hispanic/Latino; Asian/Pacific Islander; and American Indian/Alaskan Native.

BEGINNINGS for Parents of Children Who Are Deaf or Hard of Hearing

Internet: http://www.beginningssvcs.com
The Beginnings website provides a well-balanced, overview of information that is important for families with deaf children. Information about early intervention, communication options, the hearing system and hearing loss, technology, and laws related to children with hearing loss is included.

Bibliography

Allen, T., Rawlings, B. W., & Remington, E. (1993). Demographic and audiological profiles of children with cochlear implants. *American Annals of the Deaf, 138,* 260–266.

Allum, D. J. (1996). Basics of cochlear implant systems. In D. J. Allum (Ed.), *Cochlear implant rehabilitation in children and adults* (pp. 1–21). San Diego: Singular.

Bailey, D. (1996). Foreword. In P. Beckman (Ed.), *Strategies for working with families of young children with disabilities* (p. xii). Baltimore: Brookes.

Balkany, T. (1995). The rescuers. In A. S. Uziel & M. Mondain (Eds.), *Advances in Oto-Rhino-Laryngology: Vol. 50. Cochlear implants in children* (pp. 4–8). Basel: Karger.

Bess, F. H. (1985). The minimally hearing-impaired child. *Ear and Hearing, 6*(1), 43–47.

Bess, F. H., Dodd-Murphy, J., & Parker, R. A. (1998). Children with minimal sensorineural hearing loss: Prevalence, educational performance, and functional status. *Ear and Hearing, 19*(5), 339–354.

Blair, J. L., Peterson, M. E., & Viehweg, S. H. (1985). The effects of mild sensorineural hearing loss on academic performance of young school-age children. *Volta Review, 87*(2), 87–93.

Bodner-Johnson, B. (1986). The family environment and achievement of deaf students: A discriminant analysis. *Exceptional Children, 52,* 443–449.

Bodner-Johnson, B., & Sass-Lehrer, M. (1999). Concepts and premises in family-school relationships. In *Sharing ideas.* Washington, DC: Laurent Clerc National Deaf Education Center, Gallaudet University.

Boyd, K., & Dunst, C. (1993). Effects of help-giving behavior on a family's sense of control and well-being. Paper presented at the 20th International Early Childhood Conference on Children with Special Needs, San Diego.

Brand, H. J., & Coetzer, M. A. (1994). Parental response to their child's hearing impairment. *Psychological Reports, 75*(3), 1363–1368.

Brasel, K. E., & Quigley, S. P. (1977). Influence of certain language and communication environments in early childhood on the development of language in deaf individuals. *Journal of Speech and Hearing Research, 20,* 81–94.

Calderon, R. (2000). Parent involvement in deaf children's education programs as a predictor of a child's language, early reading, and social-emotional development. *Journal of Deaf Studies and Deaf Education, 5,* 140–155.

Calderon, R., Bargones, J., & Sidman, S. (1998). Characteristics of hearing families and their young deaf and hard of hearing children: Early intervention follow-up. *American Annals of the Deaf, 143,* 347–362.

Calderon, R., & Greenberg, M. (1997). The effectiveness of early intervention for deaf children and children with hearing loss. In M. J. Guralnick (Ed.), *The effectiveness of early intervention.* Baltimore: Brookes.

Calderon, R., & Greenberg, M. (1999). Stress and coping in hearing mothers of children with hearing loss: Factors affecting mother and child adjustment. *American Annals of the Deaf, 144*(1), 7–18.

Calderon, R., & Greenberg, M. (2000). Challenges to parents and professionals in promoting socioemotional development in deaf children. In P. E. Spencer, C. J. Erting, & M. Marschark (Eds.), *The deaf child in the family and at school: Essays in honor of Kathryn P. Meadow-Orlans* (pp. 167–185). Mahwah, NJ: Erlbaum.

Calderon, R., & Low, S. (1998). Early social-emotional, language, and academic development in children with hearing loss: Families with and without fathers. *American Annals of the Deaf, 143,* 225–234.

Candlish, P. A. M. (1996). *Not deaf enough: Raising a child who is hard of hearing with hugs, humor, and imagination.* Washington, DC: Alexander Graham Bell Association for the Deaf and Hard of Hearing.

Carney, E. A., & Moeller, M. P. (1998). Treatment efficacy: Hearing loss in children. *Journal of Speech, Language, and Hearing Research, 41,* 561–584.

Cebe, J. (1996). Parent satisfaction with special education services in preschools. Unpublished doctoral dissertation, Gallaudet University, Washington, DC.

Cheng, L. L. (2000). Deafness: An Asian/Pacific perspective. In K. Christensen (Ed.), *Deaf plus: A multicultural perspective* (pp. 59–92). San Diego: DawnSignPress.

Christensen, K. (Ed.) (2000). *Deaf plus: A multicultural perspective.* San Diego: DawnSignPress.

Christiansen, J. B., & Leigh, I. W. (2002). *Cochlear implants in children: Ethics and choices.* Washington, DC: Gallaudet University Press.

Clark, G. M. (1999). Cochlear implants in the third millennium. *American Journal of Otology, 20,* 4–8.

Clark, G. M., Cowan, R. S. C., & Dowell, R. C. (1997). *Cochlear implantation for infants and children: Advances.* San Diego: Singular.

Cochlear Corporation. (2002). Annual report. Retrieved September 19, 2002, from http://www.cochlear.com.

Cohen, N. L. (1997). Ethical considerations regarding cochlear implants in young children. In K. Trondhjem & I. Post (Eds.), *Cochlear implants with emphasis on the pedagogical follow-up for children and adults* (pp. 37–42). Denmark: Holmens Trykkeri. Proceedings of the 17th Danavox Symposium, September 9–13, Scanticon, Kolding, Denmark.

Cohen, O., Fischgrund, J., & Redding, R. (1990). Deaf children from ethnic, linguistic, and racial minority backgrounds: An overview. *American Annals of the Deaf, 135,* 2–10.

Craig, H. B. (1992). Parent-infant education in schools for deaf children before and after PL 99-457. *American Annals of the Deaf, 137,* 69–78.

Culbertson, J. L., & Gilbert, L. E. (1986). Children with unilateral sensorineural hearing loss: Cognitive, academic, and social development. *Ear and Hearing,* 7(1), 38–42.

Dancer, J., Burl, N. T., & Waters, S. (1995). Effects of unilateral hearing loss on teacher responses to the SIFTER. *American Annals of the Deaf, 140*(3), 291–294.

Davis, J. (Ed.) (1977/1990). *Our forgotten children: Hard-of-hearing pupils in the schools.* Washington, DC: U.S. Department of Education. (Available from Self-Help for Hard of Hearing People, 7800 Wisconsin Ave., Bethesda, MD 20814.)

Davis, J. M., Elfenbein, J., Schum, R., & Bentler, R. A. (1986). Effects of mild and moderate hearing impairments on language, educational, and psychosocial behavior of children. *Journal of Speech and Hearing Disorders, 51,* 53–62.

Desselle, D. (1994). Self-esteem, family climate, and communication patterns in relation to deafness. *American Annals of the Deaf, 139,* 322–328.

Diefendorf, A. O. (1988). Behavioral evaluation of hearing-impaired children. In F. H. Bess (Ed.), *Hearing impairment in children* (pp. 133–151). Parkton, MD: York Press.

Downs, M. P. (1974). Deafness management quotient (DMQ). *Hearing and Speech News, 42,* 26–28.

Downs, M. P. (1995). Contribution of mild hearing loss to auditory language learning problems. In R. J. Roesser & M. P. Downs (Eds.), *Auditory disorders in school children* (3rd ed., pp. 189–200). New York: Thieme Medical.

Dunst, C. J., Jenkins, V., & Trivette, C. M. (1984). Family support scale: Reliability and validity. *Journal of Individual, Family, and Community Wellness, 7,* 45–52.

Eleweke, C. J., & Rodda, M. (2000). Factors contributing to parents' selection of a communication mode to use with their deaf children. *American Annals of the Deaf, 145,* 375–383.

Erting, C. J., Prezioso, C., & Hynes, M. O. (1994). The interactional context of deaf mother-infant communication. In V. Volterra and C. J. Erting (Eds.), *From gesture to language in hearing and deaf children* (pp. 97–106). Washington, DC: Gallaudet University Press.

Erting, C. J., Thumann-Prezioso, C., & Benedict, B. S. (2000). Bilingualism in a deaf family: Fingerspelling in early childhood. In P. E. Spencer, C. J. Erting, and M. Marschark (Eds.), *The deaf child in the family and at school: Essays in honor of Kathryn P. Meadow-Orlans* (pp. 41–54). Mahwah, NJ: Erlbaum.

Fenson, L., Dale, P., Reznick, S., Bates, E., Thal, D., Hartung, J., & Reilly, J. (1991). *Technical manual for the MacArthur Communicative Development Inventories.* Developmental Psychology Laboratories, San Diego State University.

Francis, H. W., Koch, M. E., Wyatt, J. R., & Niparko, J. K. (1999). Trends in educational placement and cost-benefit considerations in children with cochlear implants. *Archives of Otolaryngological Head Neck Surgery, 125,* 499–505.

Gallaudet Research Institute. (2001). Regional and national summary report of data from the 1999–2000 Annual Survey of Deaf and Hard of Hearing Children and Youth. Washington, DC: Gallaudet University.

Geer, S. (1985). Family law: Issues raised by deafness. *Gallaudet Today, 15,* 11.

Geers, A. E., & Moog, J. S. (1987). Predicting spoken language acquisition in profoundly deaf children. *Journal of Speech and Hearing Disorders, 52,* 84–94.

Geers, A. E., & Moog, J. S. (1992). Speech perception and production skills of students with impaired hearing from oral and total communication education settings. *Journal of Speech and Hearing Research, 35,* 1384–1393.

Geers, A. E., & Moog, J. S. (1995). Assessing the benefits of cochlear implants in an oral education program. In A. S. Uziel & M. Mondain (Eds.), *Advances in oto-rhino-laryngology: Vol. 50. Cochlear implants in children* (pp. 119–124). Basel: Karger.

Gerner de Garcia, B. (2000). Meeting the needs of Hispanic/Latino deaf students. In K. M. Christensen (Ed.), *Deaf plus: A multicultural perspective* (pp. 149–198). San Diego: DawnSignPress.

Gerner de Garcia, B. (1993). Addressing the needs of Hispanic deaf children. In K. M. Christensen and G. L. Delgado (Eds.), *Multicultural issues in deafness* (pp. 91–112). White Plains, NY: Longman.

Giangreco, M. F., Cloninger, C. J., Mueller, P. H., Yuan, S., & Ashworth, S. (1991). Perspectives of parents whose children have dual sensory impairments. *Journal of the Association for Persons with Severe Handicaps, 16*(1), 14–24.

Giangreco, M. F., Edelman, S. W., MacFarland, S., & Luiselli, T. E. (1997). Attitudes about education and related service provision for students with deaf-blindness and multiple disabilities. *Exceptional Children, 63*(3), 329–342.

Gilhool, T. K., & Gran, J. A. (1985). Legal rights of disabled parents. In S. K. Thurman (Ed.), *Children of handicapped parents: Research and clinical perspectives* (pp. 11–34). Orlando: Academic Press.

Greenberg, M. T., Calderon, R., & Kusché, C. (1984). Early intervention using simultaneous communication with deaf infants: The effects on communication development. *Child Development, 55,* 607–616.

Greenberg, M. T., & Crnic, K. A. (1988). Longitudinal predictors of developmental status and social interaction in premature and full-term infants at age two. *Child Development, 59,* 554–570.

Greenberg, M. T., & Kusché, C. A. (1993). *Promoting social and emotional development in deaf children: The PATHS project.* Seattle: University of Washington.

Gregory, S. (1995). *Deaf children and their families.* Cambridge: Cambridge University Press.

Harrison, M., Darnhardt, M., & Roush, J. (1996). Families' perceptions of early intervention services for children with hearing loss. *Language, Speech, and Hearing Services in Schools, 27,* 203–214.

Harrison, M., & Roush, J. (1996). Age of suspicion, identification, and intervention for infants and young children with hearing loss: A national survey. *Ear and Hearing, 17,* 55–62.

Harvey, M. A. (1989). *Psychotherapy with deaf and hard-of-hearing persons: A systemic model.* Hillsdale, NJ: Erlbaum.

Hasenstab, M. S. (1997). Cognitive performance in children using multichannel cochlear implants. In K. Trondhjem & I. Post (Eds.), *Cochlear implants with emphasis on the pedagogical follow-up for children and adults* (pp. 115–136). Denmark: Holmens Trykkeri. Proceedings of the 17th Danavox Symposium, September 9–13, Scanticon, Kolding, Denmark.

Hauser-Cram, P., Warfield, M. E., Shonkoff, J., & Krauss, M. W. (2001). Children with disabilities: A longitudinal study of child development and parent well-being. *Monograph of the Society for Research in Child Development, 66*(3, Serial No. 266).

Hernandez, D. J. (1997). Child development and the social demography of childhood. *Child Development, 68,* 149–169.

Hindley, P. (2000). Child and adolescent psychiatry. In P. Hindley & N. Kitson (Eds.), *Mental health and deafness* (pp. 42–74). London: Whurr.

Hintermair, M. (2000a). Children who are hearing impaired with additional disabilities and related aspects of parental stress. *Exceptional Children, 66*(3), 327–332.

Hintermair, M. (2000b). Hearing impairment, social networks, and coping: The need for families with hearing-impaired children to relate to other parents and to hearing-impaired adults. *American Annals of the Deaf, 145*(1), 41–53.

Holden-Pitt, L. (1997). A look at residential school placement patterns for students from deaf- and hearing-parented families. *American Annals of the Deaf, 142,* 108–114.

Holden-Pitt, L., & Diaz, J. A. (1998). Thirty years of the annual survey of deaf and hard-of-hearing children and youth: A glance over the decades. *American Annals of the Deaf, 143*(2), 72–76.

Jamison, J. R. (1994). Instructional discourse strategies: Differences between hearing and deaf mothers of deaf children. *First Language, 14,* 153–171.

Johnson, R. E., Liddell, S., & Erting, C. (1989). *Unlocking the curriculum: Principles for achieving access in deaf education.* Gallaudet Research Institute Working Occasional Paper Series, 89–93. Washington, DC: Gallaudet Research Institute.

Jones, T. W., & Jones, J. K. (in press). Challenges in educating young children with multiple disabilities. In B. Bodner-Johnson & M. Sass-Lehrer (Eds.), *Early edu-*

cation for deaf and hard of hearing toddlers and their families: Integrating best practices and future perspectives. Baltimore: Brookes.

Kampfe, C. M., Harrison, M., Oettinger, T., Luddington, J., McDonald-Bell, C., & Pillsbury, H. C. (1993). Parental expectations as a factor in evaluating children for the multichannel cochlear implant. *American Annals of the Deaf, 138,* 297–303.

Kluwin, T. N., & Gaustad, M. G. (1991). Predicting family communication choices. *American Annals of the Deaf, 136,* 28–34.

Kluwin, T. N., & Stewart, D. A. (2000). Cochlear implants for younger children: A preliminary description of the parental decision process and outcomes. *American Annals of the Deaf, 145*(1), 26–35.

Koester, L. S., & Meadow-Orlans, K. P. (1990). Parenting a deaf child: Stress, strength, and support. In D. F. Moores & K. P. Meadow-Orlans (Eds.), *Educational and developmental aspects of deafness* (pp. 299–320). Washington, DC: Gallaudet University Press.

Kovach, J., & Jacks, R. (1989). Program evaluation using the Dakota Project Parent Satisfaction Survey: A manual for administration and interpretation of findings using a validated instrument. Eagan, MN: Dakota.

Krauss, M. W., Upshur, C. C., Shonkoff, J. P., & Hauser-Cram, P. (1993). The impact of parent groups on mothers of infants with disabilities. *Journal of Early Intervention, 17*(1), 8–20.

Lane, H. (1992). *The mask of benevolence.* New York: Knopf.

Lane, H., Hoffmeister, R., & Bahan, B. (1996). *A journey into the deaf world.* San Diego: DawnSignPress.

Lane, S., Bell, L., & Parson-Tylka, T. (1997). *My turn to learn: A communication guide for parents of deaf or hard of hearing children.* Surrey, BC, Canada: Elks Family Hearing Resource Centre.

Ling, D. (1989). *Foundations of spoken language for hearing-impaired children.* Washington, DC: Alexander Graham Bell Association for the Deaf and Hard of Hearing.

Luterman, D. (1987). *Deafness in the family.* Boston: Little Brown.

Luterman, D. (1999). *The young deaf child.* Baltimore: York Press.

Luterman, D., & Kurtzer-White, E. (1999). Identifying hearing loss: Parents' needs. *American Journal of Audiology,* 13–18.

Lynas, W. (1999). Communication options. In J. Stokes (Ed.), *Hearing impaired infants: Support in the first eighteen months* (pp. 98–128). Baltimore: Brookes.

MacKenzie, K. (Ed.). (1999). *Starting point: A resource for parents of deaf or hard of hearing children.* Toronto: Canadian Hearing Society.

Mapp, I., & Hudson, R. (1997). Stress and coping among African American and Hispanic parents of deaf children. *American Annals of the Deaf, 142*(1), 48–56.

Marschark, M. (1997). *Raising and educating a deaf child.* New York: Oxford University Press.

Marschark, M. (2000). Language development in children who are deaf and hard of hearing: A research synthesis and implications for policy and practice. Unpublished manuscript prepared for Project FORUM at the National Association of State Directors of Special Education (NASDSE).

Marschark, M., Lang, H. G., & Albertini, J. A. (2002). *Educating deaf students: From research to practice.* New York: Oxford University Press.

McWilliam, P. J., Winton, P., & Crais, E. (1996). *Practical strategies for family-centered intervention.* San Diego: Singular.

Meadow, K. P. (1968). Early manual communication in relation to the deaf child's intellectual, social, and communicative skills. *American Annals of the Deaf, 113,* 29–41.

Meadow, K. P., Greenberg, M. T., & Erting, C. (1985). Attachment behavior of deaf children with deaf parents. In S. Chess and A. Thomas (Eds.), *Annual progress in child psychiatry and child development, 1984* (pp. 176–187). New York: Brunner/Mazel.

Meadow, K. P., Greenberg, M. T., Erting, C., & Carmichael, H. (1981). Interactions of deaf mothers and deaf preschool children: Comparisons with three other groups of deaf and hearing dyads. *American Annals of the Deaf, 126,* 454–468.

Meadow–Orlans, K. P. (1983). An instrument for assessment of social–emotional adjustment in hearing-impaired preschoolers. *American Annals of the Deaf, 128,* 826–834.

Meadow–Orlans, K. P. (1984). Social adjustment of preschool children: Deaf and hearing, with and without other handicaps. *Topics in Early Childhood Special Education, 3,* 27–40.

Meadow–Orlans, K. P. (1987). An analysis of the effectiveness of early intervention programs for hearing-impaired children. In M. J. Guralnick & F. C. Bennett (Eds.), *The effectiveness of early intervention for at-risk and handicapped children* (pp. 325–362). New York: Academic Press.

Meadow-Orlans, K. P. (1990). The impact of childhood hearing loss on the family. In D. F. Moores & K. P. Meadow-Orlans (Eds.), *Educational and developmental aspects of deafness* (pp. 321–338). Washington, DC: Gallaudet University Press.

Meadow-Orlans, K. P. (1997). Effects of mother and infant hearing status on interactions at twelve and eighteen months. *Journal of Deaf Studies and Deaf Education, 2,* 26–36.

Meadow-Orlans, K. P. (2001). Research and deaf education: Moving ahead while glancing back. *Journal of Deaf Studies and Deaf Education, 6,* 143–148.

Meadow-Orlans, K. P. (2002a). Parenting with a sensory or physical disability. In M. H. Bornstein (Ed.), *Handbook of parenting* (Vol. 4, 2nd ed., pp. 259–293). Mahwah, NJ: Erlbaum.

Meadow-Orlans, K. P. (2002b). Social change and conflict: Context for research on deafness. In M. D. Clark, M. Marschark, & M. Karchmer (Eds.), *Language, speech and social-emotional development of children who are deaf or hard of hearing: Context, cognition, and deafness* (pp. 161–178). Washington, DC: Gallaudet University Press.

Meadow-Orlans, K. P. (in press). Support for parents of deaf and hard of hearing children: Promoting visual attention and literacy in a changing world. In B. Bodner-Johnson & M. Sass-Lehrer (Eds.), *Early education for deaf and hard of hearing infants and toddlers and their families.* Baltimore: Brookes.

Meadow-Orlans, K. P., & Sass-Lehrer, M. (1995). Support services for families of children who are deaf: Challenges for professionals. *Topics in Early Childhood Special Education 15*(3), 314–334.

Meadow-Orlans, K. P., Sass-Lehrer, M., & Mertens, D. M. (2000, July). Parent to parent: Advice for parents with young deaf or hard of hearing children. Paper presented at the American Society for Deaf Children, Washington, DC.

Meadow-Orlans, K. P., Smith-Gray, S., & Dyssegaard, B. (1995). Infants who are deaf or hard of hearing, with and without physical/cognitive disabilities. *American Annals of the Deaf, 140*(3), 279–286.

Meadow-Orlans, K. P., & Steinberg, A. G. (1993). Effects of infant hearing loss and maternal support on mother-infant interactions at eighteen months. *Journal of Applied Developmental Psychology, 14,* 407–426.

Mertens, D. M. (1998). *Research methods in education and psychology: Integrating diversity.* Thousand Oaks, CA: Sage.

Mertens, D. M., & McLaughlin, J. (1995). *Research methods in special education.* Thousand Oaks, CA: Sage.

Mertens, D. M., Sass-Lehrer, M., & Scott-Olson, K. (2000). Sensitivity in the family-professional relationship: Parental experiences in families with young deaf and hard of hearing children. In P. E. Spencer, C. Erting, & M. Marschark (Eds.), *The deaf child in the family and at school.* Mahwah, NJ: Erlbaum.

Meyer, T. A., Svirsky, M. A., Kirk, K., & Miyamoto, R. T. (1998). Improvements in speech perception by children with profound prelingual hearing loss: Effects of device, communication mode, and chronological age. *Journal of Speech, Language, and Hearing Research, 41,* 846–858.

Miyamoto, R. T., Osberger, M. J., Robbins, A. M., Myres, W. A., & Kessler, K. (1993). Prelingually deafened children's performance with the nucleus multi-channel cochlear implant. *American Journal of Otology, 14,* 437–445.

Moeller, M. P. (2000). Early intervention and language development in children who are deaf and hard of hearing. *Pediatrics, 106,*(3), E43.

Moeller, M. P., & Condon, M. (1994). D.E.I.P.: A collaborative problem-solving approach to early intervention. In J. Roush & N. Matkin (Eds.), *Infants and toddlers with hearing loss: Family-centered assessment and intervention.* Baltimore: York Press.

Mohay, H. (2000). Language in sight: Mothers' strategies for making language visually accessible to deaf children. In P. E. Spencer, C. Erting, & M. Marschark (Eds.), *The deaf child in the family and at school.* Mahwah, NJ: Erlbaum.

Moores, D. F. (2000). Editorial: How's that again? *American Annals of the Deaf, 145,* 3.

Moores, D. F. (2001). *Educating the deaf: Psychology, principles, and practices* (5th ed.). Boston: Houghton Mifflin.

Moses, K. L. (1985). Infant deafness and parental grief: Psychosocial early intervention. In F. Powell, T. Finitzo-Heber, S. Friel-Patti, & D. Henderson (Eds.), *Education of the hearing-impaired child* (pp. 86–102). San Diego: College-Hill Press.

Mowl, G. E. (1996). Raising deaf children in a hearing society: Struggles and challenges for deaf native ASL signers. In I. Parasnis (Ed.), *Cultural and language diversity and the deaf experience* (pp. 232–245). New York: Cambridge University Press.

National Association of the Deaf (NAD) Cochlear Implant Committee. (2001). NAD position statement on cochlear implants. *NAD Broadcaster, 23,* 14–15.

National Center for Hearing Assessment and Management. (2002). Retrieved September 21, 2002, from http://www.infanthearing.org.

Nevins, M. E., & Chute, P. M. (1996). *Children with cochlear implants in educational settings.* San Diego: Singular.

Niskar, A. S., Kieszak, S. M., Holmes, A., Esteban, E., Rubin, C., & Brody, D. J. (1998). Prevalence of hearing loss among children 6 to 19 years of age. *Journal of the American Medical Association, 179*(14), 1071–1075.

O'Donoghue, G. M. (1996). Cochlear implants in children: Principles, practice and predictions. *Journal of the Royal Society of Medicine, 89,* 345P–347P.

Ogden, P. (1996). *The silent garden: Raising your deaf child* (2nd ed.). Washington, DC: Gallaudet University Press.

Padden, C. A. (1996). From the cultural to the bicultural: The modern deaf community. In I. Parasnis (Ed.), *Cultural and language diversity and the deaf experience* (pp. 79–98). Cambridge: Cambridge University Press.

Padden, C., & Humphries, T. (1988). *Deaf in America: Voices from a culture.* Cambridge: Harvard University Press.

Paul, P., & Quigley, S. (1990). *Education and deafness.* New York: Longman.

Pipp-Siegel, S., Blair, N. L., Deas, A. M., Pressman, L. J., & Yoshinaga-Itano, C. (1999). Touch and emotional availability in hearing and deaf or hard of hearing toddlers and their hearing mothers. *Volta Review, 100*(5), 279–298.

Pipp-Siegel, S., Sedey, A. L., & Yoshinaga-Itana, C. (2002). Predictors of parental stress of mothers of young children with hearing loss. *Journal of Deaf Studies and Deaf Education, 7,* 1–17.

Powers, A. R., Elliott, R. N., Patterson, D., Shaw, S., & Taylor, C. (1995). Family environment and deaf and hard-of-hearing students with mild additional disabilities. *Journal of Childhood Communication Disorders, 17*(1), 15–19.

Preston, P. (1994). *Mother father deaf: Living between sound and silence.* Cambridge: Harvard University Press.

Quittner, A. L., Steck, J. T., & Rouiller, R. L. (1991). Cochlear implants in children: A study of parental stress and adjustment. *American Journal of Otology, 12* (Suppl.), 95–104.

Ramsey, C. (2000). On the border: Cultures, families, and schooling in a transnational region. In K. Christensen (Ed.), *Deaf plus: A multicultural perspective* (pp. 121–148). San Diego: DawnSignPress.

Ritter-Brinton, K., & Stewart, D. (1992). Hearing parents and deaf children: Some perspectives on sign communication and service delivery. *American Annals of the Deaf, 137,* 85–91.

Rizer, F. M., & Burkey, J. M. (1999). Cochlear implantation in the very young child. *Otolaryngologic Clinics of North America, 32,* 1117–1125.

Rodriguez, O., & Santiviago, M. (1991). Hispanic deaf adolescents: A cultural minority. *Volta Review, 93*(5), 89–97.

Roland, P. S. (1995). Medical aspects of disorders of the auditory system. In R. J. Roesser & M. P. Downs (Eds.), *Auditory disorders in school children* (3rd ed., pp. 56–75). New York: Thieme Medical.

Rosenbaum, J. (2000, March). *Family functioning and child behavior: Impacts of communication in hearing families with a deaf child.* (Publication number 3038026) Washington, DC: Gallaudet University.

Ross, M. (1990). Definitions and descriptions. In J. Davis (Ed.), *Our forgotten children: Hard-of-hearing pupils in the schools* (pp. 3–18). Washington, DC: U.S. Department of Education.

Roush, J., Harrison, M., & Palsha, S. (1991). Family-centered early intervention: The perceptions of professionals. *American Annals of the Deaf, 136,* 360–366.

Roush, J., Harrison, M., Palsha, S., & Davidson, D. (1992). A national survey of educational preparation programs for early intervention specialists. *American Annals of the Deaf, 137,* 425–430.

Sandall, S., McLean, M., & Smith, B. (2000). *DEC recommended practices in early intervention/early childhood special education.* Longmont, CO: Sopris West.

Sass-Lehrer, M., & Bodner-Johnson, B. (1989). Public Law 99-457: A new challenge to early intervention. *American Annals of the Deaf, 134,* 71–77.

Sass-Lehrer, M., Meadow-Orlans, K., Mertens, D., & Scott-Olson, K. (1999, July). Families with young hard of hearing children. Paper presented at the 59th biennial conference of the Convention of American Instructors of the Deaf, Los Angeles.

Sass-Lehrer, M., Meadow-Orlans, K., Mertens, D., Scott-Olson, K., & Steinmetz, S. (1999, May). Hearing and deaf parents of young deaf children: Challenges and advice. Paper presented at the National Symposium on Childhood Deafness, Sioux Falls, SD.

Schein, J. D. (1996). The demography of deafness. In P. C. Higgins & J. E. Nash (Eds.), *Understanding deafness socially* (2nd ed., pp. 21–43). Springfield, IL: Thomas.

Schildroth, A. N., & Hotto, S. A. (1993). Annual survey of hearing-impaired children and youth: 1991–1992 school year. *American Annals of the Deaf, 138,* 163–171.

Schildroth, A. N., & Hotto, S. A. (1996). Changes in student and program characteristics, 1984–1985 and 1994–1995. *American Annals of the Deaf, 141,* 68–71.

Schlesinger, H. S. (1992). The elusive X factor: Parental contributions to literacy. In M. Walworth, D. F. Moores, & T. J. O'Rourke (Eds.), *A free hand: Enfranchising the education of deaf children* (pp. 37–64). Silver Spring, MD: TJ.

Schwartz, S. (Ed.). (1996). *Choices in deafness: A parent's guide to communication options* (2nd ed.). Baltimore: Woodbine House.

Searls, S. C., & Johnston, D. R. (1996). Growing up deaf in deaf families: Two different experiences. In I. Parasnis (Ed.), *Cultural and language diversity and the deaf experience* (pp. 201–224). Cambridge: Cambridge University Press.

Shonkoff, J. P., Hauser-Cram, P., Krauss, M. W., & Upshur, C. C. (1992). Development of infants with disabilities and their families. *Monographs of the Society for Research in Child Development, 57*(6, Serial No. 230).

Singer, G. H. S., Marquis, J., Powers, L. K., Blanchard, L., Divenere, N., Santelli, B., Ainbinder, J. G., & Sharp, M. (1999). A multisite evaluation of parent-to-parent programs for parents of children with disabilities. *Journal of Early Intervention, 22*(3), 217–229.

Spencer, L. J., Tye-Murray, N., & Tomblin, J. B. (1998). The production of English inflectional morphology, speech production, and listening performance in children with cochlear implants. *Ear and Hearing, 19,* 310–318.

Spencer, P. E. (2000a). Every opportunity: A case study of hearing parents and their deaf child. In P. Spencer, C. Erting, & M. Marschark (Eds.), *The deaf child at home and at school.* Mahwah, NJ: Erlbaum.

Spencer, P. E. (2000b). Looking without listening: Is audition a prerequisite for normal development of visual attention during infancy? *Journal of Deaf Studies and Deaf Education, 5,* 291–302.

Spencer, P. E. (2002). Language development of children with cochlear Implants. In J. B. Christiansen & I. W. Leigh (Eds.), *Cochlear implants in children: Ethics and choices* (pp. 222–249). Washington, DC: Gallaudet University Press.

Spencer, P. E., Christiansen, J. B., & Leigh, I. W. (2002). History of cochlear implants. In J. B. Christiansen & I. W. Leigh (Eds.), *Cochlear implants in children: Ethics and choices* (pp. 15–44). Washington, DC: Gallaudet University Press.

Steinberg, A., & Bain, L. (2001). Parental decision making for infants with hearing impairment. *International Pediatrics, 6,* 1–6.

Steinberg, A., Brainsky, A., Bain, L., Montoya, L., Indenbaum, M., & Potsic, W. (2000). Parental values in the decision about cochlear implantation. *International Journal of Pediatric Otorhinolaryngology, 55,* 99–107.

Steinberg, A., Davila, J. R., Collazo, J., Loew, R. C., & Fischgrund, J. E. (1997). "A little sign and a lot of love . . . ": Attitudes, perceptions, and beliefs of Hispanic families with deaf children. *Qualitative Health Research* 7(2), 202–222.

Stredler-Brown, A. (1998). Early intervention for infants and toddlers who are deaf and hard of hearing: New perspectives. *Journal of Educational Audiology, 6,* 45–49.

Stredler-Brown, A., & Arehart, K. H. (2000). Universal newborn hearing screening: Impact on early intervention services. In C. Yoshinaga-Itano & A. Sedey (Eds.), Language, speech and social-emotional development of children who are deaf or hard of hearing: The early years [Monograph]. *Volta Review, 100*(5), 85–117.

Stuckless, E. R., & Birch, J. W. (1966). The influence of early manual communication on the linguistic development of deaf children. *American Annals of the Deaf, 111,* 452–460; 499–504.

Szagun, G. (2000). The acquisition of grammatical and lexical structures in children with cochlear implants: A developmental psycholinguistic approach. *Audiology & Neuro-Otology, 5,* 39–47.

Todd, N. W. (1986). High-risk populations for otitis media. In J. F. Kavanagh (Ed.), *Otitis media and child development* (pp. 52–69). Parkton, MD: York Press.

Tolland, A. M. (1995). Diagnosis: Hearing loss. Mothering a child with hearing loss. *Hearing Loss: The Journal of Self-Help for Hard of Hearing People, 16*(4), 12–17.

Tomblin, J. B., Spencer, L., Flock, S., Tyler, R., & Gantz, B. (1999). A comparison of language achievement in children with cochlear implants and children using hearing aids. *Journal of Speech, Language, and Hearing Research, 42,* 497–511.

Tonelson, S., & Watkins, S. (1979). The SKI★HI Language Development Scale. Logan: SKI★HI Institute, Utah State University.

Tye-Murray, N., & Kelsay, D. M. R. (1993). A communication training program for parents of cochlear implant users. *Volta Review, 95,* 21–31.

U.S. Census Bureau. (2001). Census 2000 shows America's diversity. Washington, DC: Author. CB01-CN.61.

Vacarri, C., & Marschark, M. (1997). Communication between parents and deaf children: Implications for social-emotional development. *Journal of Child Psychiatry, 18*(7), 793–801.

Vernon, M., & Koh, S. D. (1970). Early manual communication and deaf children's achievement. *American Annals of the Deaf, 115,* 527–536.

Wathum-Ocama, J. C. (2000). Attitudes of parents of Hmong deaf or hard of hearing students: An ethnographic study. *Dissertation Abstracts International, 60,* 8A, March 2000, 2803 (University Microfilms International).

Watkins, S., Pittman, P., & Walden, B. (1998). The deaf mentor experimental project for young children who are deaf and their families. *American Annals of the Deaf, 143,*(1), 29–34.

Wills, R. (1998). Children with mild and moderate hearing losses. In J. Stokes (Ed.), *Hearing-impaired infants: The first eighteen months* (pp. 80–97). London: Whurr.

Wolfe, V. (2001). A look at rural families: Weighing educational options. In *Sharing results.* Washington, DC: Laurent Clerc National Deaf Education Center, Gallaudet University.

Wolff, A. B., & Harkins, J. E. (1986). Multihandicapped students. In A. N. Schildroth & M. A. Karchmer (Eds.), *Deaf children in America* (pp. 55–83). San Diego: College-Hill.

Yoshinaga-Itano, C. (2000). Successful outcomes for deaf and hard of hearing children. *Seminars in Hearing, 21,* 309–325.

Yoshinaga-Itano, C., & Marion Downs Center for Infant Hearing. (2001, July). Infant hearing systems: Assuring quality outcomes. Paper presented at the Florida State Symposium on Early Identification and Intervention, St. Augustine.

Yoshinaga-Itano, C., & Sedey, A. (2000). Early speech development in children who are deaf or hard of hearing: Interrelationships with language and hearing. In C. Yoshinaga-Itano and A. Sedey (Eds.), Language, speech, and social-emotional development of children who are deaf or hard of hearing: The early years [Monograph]. *Volta Review, 100,* (5), 181–211.

Yoshinaga-Itano, C., Sedey, A. L., Coulter, C. K., & Mehl, A. L. (1998). Language of early- and later-identified children with hearing loss. *Pediatrics, 102*(5), 1161–1171.

Young, A. (1997). Conceptualizing parents' sign language use in bilingual early intervention. *Journal of Deaf Studies and Deaf Education, 2,* 264–276.

Author Index

Subject Index